STUDY GUIDE TO ACCOMPANY

Fundamental Skills and Concepts in Patient Care

Seventh Edition

BARBARA R. STRIGHT, PH.D, R.N.

Associate Professor
School of Nursing
Clarion University of Pennsylvania

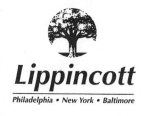

Lippincott

Philadelphia • New York • Baltimore

Ancillary Editor: Doris S. Wray
Senior Production Manager: Helen Ewan
Composition: Shepherd, Inc.
Printer/Binder: Victor Graphics

9th Edition

ISBN: 0-7817-2317-5

The material contained in this volume was submitted as previously unpublished material, except in the instances in which credit has been given to the source from which some of the illustrative material was derived.

Any procedure or practice described in this book should be applied by the health care practitioner under appropriate supervision in accordance with professional standards of care used with regard to the unique circumstances that apply in each practice situation. Care has been taken to confirm the accuracy of information presented and to describe generally accepted practices. However, the authors, editors, and publisher cannot accept any responsibility for errors or omissions or for any consequences from application of the information in this book and make no warranty express or implied, with respect to the contents of the book.

The authors and publisher have exerted every effort to ensure that drug selection and dosage set forth in this text are in accordance with current recommendations and practice at the time of publication. However, in view of ongoing research, changes in government regulations, and the constant flow of information relating to drug therapy and drug reactions, the reader is urged to check the package insert for each drug for any change in indications and dosage and for added warnings and precautions. This is particularly important when the recommended agent is a new or infrequently employed drug.

9 8 7 6 5 4 3 2 1

Dedication

This work is dedicated to my Bunny Boy with love and gratitude for his patience and understanding while I worked.

Preface

This study guide has been prepared in conjunction with the textbook *Fundamental Skills and Concepts in Patient Care,* seventh edition. The two books are correlated chapter by chapter. The study guide is ideally suited to be used with the textbook. However, it also can be used with other texts, or it can be used by anyone interested in examining his or her knowledge of basic skills in patient care without reference to a specific text.

The primary purpose of this study guide is to offer tools so that the student can evaluate fundamental knowledge and skills that are considered important in the practice of nursing. Each chapter begins with a summary statement of learning objectives. These are followed by examination items and other exercises designed to test the objectives.

Attempting to test everything related to a particular body of knowledge is an impractical and impossible goal. As is true of all evaluation tools, those in this study guide sample relevant material. If the reader believes certain material was omitted that should have been included, the study guide can be used as a guide to develop similar tools for particular situations.

This study guide contains matching, multiple choice, true or false, and short answer questions, and performance checklists, and critical thinking exercises when appropriate.

Answers to the multiple choice, true or false, matching, and short answer are provided at the end of the study guide. The correct answer and rationale are given for each item along with the page number, skill, or table in *Fundamental Skills and Concepts in Patient Care,* seventh edition, where answers can be verified. Answers are not provided for the critical thinking exercises since these questions are mainly subjective and for discussion and expansion purposes.

The performance checklists offer an opportunity for students to examine their techniques when giving care. Students may complete the forms themselves, or they may select an observer to complete the form for them. There is space provided for comments where notes can be made about what further practice is indicated, what errors were made, or suggestions that will help improve performance. It is intended that these forms be completed during or immediately after patient care is given. However, many could be used in laboratory situations when students are practicing skills before giving care to patients. There are no correct answers to these forms because they apply to specific care.

The chapters in Units I through III deal with basic information that nurses use whenever they care for patients, regardless of each patient's specific needs. Units IV through XII present nursing skills required in specific areas of patient care, that is, health maintenance and promotion, changing levels of wellness, health restoration, and death and dying.

The pages of this study guide are perforated. The examinations may be removed if this proves convenient. Instructors may wish to remove the correct answers and rationales and then return them for each chapter as students complete their self-testing. The performance checklists may be removed for review and discussion.

The primary objective of this study guide will have been met when the student is able to use basic nursing skills with confidence.

To the Student

The primary purpose of this study guide is to offer tools for you to evaluate your mastery of the fundamental knowledge and skills that are considered important in the practice of nursing. The study guide is correlated chapter by chapter with *Fundamental Skills and Concepts in Patient Care,* seventh edition.

Each chapter begins with a summary of the content of the relevant text chapter and a list of learning objectives. These are followed by examination items and other exercises designed to test your achievement of these objectives.

Included are multiple choice, true or false, and short answer questions, as well as matching, and discussion questions and performance checklists.

Answers to multiple choice, true or false, matching, and short answer are provided in the Answers and Rationale section at the end of the book. Answers are not provided for the critical thinking exercises, since these are mainly subjective and are for discussion and expansion purposes.

You will have defeated part of the reason for using this study guide, however, if you look at the answers prior to working through the examinations. Also, avoid searching for clues to the correct answer among the items in each question or subsequent questions.

Sometimes it may be relatively quick and easy to rule out one or two choices as incorrect. Then concentrate on the remaining choices. Narrowing your options sharpens your thinking by placing attention on choices you believe are reasonably correct.

Be sure to read each item carefully. Watch for key words such as *best, least, rarely, primarily,* and *con-*

traindicated. When key words are overlooked, there is often no basis for selecting a correct answer.

Use only the information you are given. Do not attempt to read additional information into an item or make assumptions about it.

Pace yourself occasionally. Select a certain number of items and plan to spend an average of about one minute on each item. If you are doing well, slow your speed; if you are falling behind, try to work faster. This type of practice helps prepare you for timed examinations such as the state licensing examinations.

After learning which items you have answered incorrectly, go back and study them again. Also study the items you answered correctly to see whether you understand the information on which it was based, Concentrate on *understanding* the information, rather than memorizing it.

The examinations do not have a passing or failing score. If all or nearly all items are answered correctly, you probably have mastered the chapter's content. If you fail to give correct answers to at least 80% to 90% of the items, review is suggested. You should seriously question whether you have mastered the content of a chapter if you fail to answer at least 80% of the items correctly.

The performance checklists contain directions concerning their use. You may examine your own nursing practice, or you may wish to ask another person to evaluate you. After the forms are completed, you should know which skills you have mastered and what further study is indicated.

Acknowledgments

The author wishes to thank the following people and the agencies for which they work for their help in preparing this text.

- Doris Wray, for her advice, support, assistance and encouragement during the preparation of this edition.
- The nursing students of Clarion University of Pennsylvania, for their encouragement, suggestions, and assistance in pointing out errors in the previous edition of this study guide.

Contents

CHAPTER 1

Nursing Foundations

SUMMARY

Nursing is one of the youngest professions but one of the oldest arts. It evolved from the familial roles of nurturing and care taking. Early responsibilities included: assisting women during childbirth, suckling healthy newborns, and ministering to the ill, aged, and helpless within the household and surrounding community. Its hallmark was caring more than curing.

Chapter 1 traces the historical development of nursing from its unorganized beginning to current practice. Ironically, nursing is returning to the community-based practice from which it originated.

MATCHING QUESTIONS

Directions: For items 1 through 4, match the theorists in Part B with the theories in Part A.

Part A

C 1. ___a___ The Adaptation Theory
A 2. ___B___ The Environmental Theory
D 3. ___D___ The Self-Care Theory
B 4. ___C___ The Basic Needs Theory

Part B

a. Florence Nightingale
b. Virginia Henderson
c. Sister Callista Roy
d. Dorothea Orem

Directions: For items 5 through 8, match the definitions in Part B with the skills in Part A.

Part A

5. ___D___ Assessment skills
6. ___C___ Caring skills
7. ___a___ Comforting skills
8. ___B___ Counseling skills

Part B

a. Those skills that convey security and stability during crisis
b. Those skills that involve both talking and listening
c. Those skills that restore or maintain an individual's health
d. Those skills used for interviewing, observing, and examining a patient

Directions: For items 9 through 16, match the definitions in Part B with the terms in Part A.

Part A

9. ___e___ Art
10. ___I___ Active listening
D 11. ___g___ Caring
12. ___a___ Empathy
13. ___f___ Nursing
14. ___c___ Theory
15. ___h___ Science
16. ___j___ Sympathy

Part B

a. Intuitive awareness of what the patient is experiencing
b. A personal view of oneself
c. An opinion, belief, or view that explains a process
d. The concern and attachment that occur from the close relationship of one human being with another
e. The ability to perform an act skillfully
f. The diagnosis and treatment of human responses to actual or potential health problems
g. Care intended primarily to maintain or restore physical function immediately upon admission
h. A body of knowledge unique to a particular subject
i. Hearing the content of what the patient says as well as unspoken message
j. Feeling as emotionally distraught as the patient

TRUE OR FALSE QUESTIONS

Directions: For items 1 through 7, decide if the statement is true or false and mark T or F in the space provided.

1. __T__ Nursing is one of the youngest professions yet one of the oldest arts.

2. __F__ Florence Nightingale was called into nursing after hospitals began to show evidence of improving health care.

3. __T__ Planned, consistent, and formal education was the priority of Nightingale schools while the training of American nurses was more of an unsubsidized apprenticeship.

4. __T__ The associate degree graduates are not expected to work in a management position.

5. __T__ The definition of nursing has finally stabilized after many changes.

6. __F__ Giving an abundance of "tender loving care" may delay the patient from resuming the normal activities of daily living.

7. __F__ Nurses should give advice to their patients.

MULTIPLE CHOICE QUESTIONS

Directions: For items 1 through 12, circle the letter that corresponds to the best answer for each question.

1. The service of caring for the sick changed drastically as a result of the split between King Henry VIII of England and the Catholic Church. These changes were due to which of the following:
   a. The administration of English hospitals became a duty of the state
   b. The state started hiring the ranks of criminals, widows, and orphans
   c. Nuns and priests were extradited to continental Europe
   d. The Catholic Church of England was forced to change patient care

2. Which of the following statements *best* describes how funding became available:
   a. Servicemen and their families showed their appreciation of Florence Nightingale by donating funds due to her work in Scutari
   b. Servicemen and their families supplied funding for new schools of nursing being established in the United States
   c. Florence Nightingale and her 38 volunteers proved that they could lower the infection and death rates
   d. The first Nightingale school at St. Thomas Hospital in England obtained sufficient funding to set up models for others in Europe and the United States

3. Virginia Henderson proposed which of the following definitions about nursing:
   a. The "diagnosis and treatment of human responses to actual or potential health problems"
   b. Nursing involves a special relationship and service between the nurse and those entrusted to his or her care
   c. Nursing is a human service that assists individuals to progressively maximize their self-care potential
   d. Nurses modify unhealthy aspects of the environment to put the patient in the best possible condition for nature to act

4. Which of the following theorists proposed the associate degree program in nursing: ADN
   a. Virginia Henderson
   b. Dorothea Orem
   c. Sister Callista Roy
   d. Mildred Montag

5. The Environmental Theory was developed by:
   a. Florence Nightingale
   b. Dorothea Orem
   c. Virginia Henderson
   d. Sister Callista Roy

6. Dorothea Orem's theory, as it relates to people, states that a human being is:
   a. An individual whose natural defenses are influenced by a healthy or unhealthy environment
   b. An individual with human needs that have meaning and value unique to each person
   c. An individual who utilizes self-care to sustain life and health, recover from disease or injury, or cope with its effects
   d. A social, mental, spiritual, and physical being who is affected by stimuli within his internal and external environment

7. When the nurse is using assessment skills, the primary source of information is:
   a. The patient
   b. The medical record
   c. Other health practitioners
   d. Data collected

8. The primary focus of nursing, no matter what level of care is provided for the patient, is:
   a. To give all patients "tender loving care"
   b. To give patients exactly what the doctor prescribes
   c. To be able to use complex devices and equipment
   d. To assist the patient to eventually become independent

9. Nursing skills that would be used to assist the patient in becoming an active participant in decision making are:
   a. Caring skills
   b. Counseling skills
   c. Comforting skills
   d. Assessment skills

10. Of the following, which must be understood before the nurse will be able to apply assessment skills to predict which nursing interventions are most appropriate for producing the desired outcome:
    a. Nursing science
    b. Nursing arts
    c. Nursing diagnosis
    d. Nursing theories

11. The most recent definition of nursing was developed by:
    a. The International Council of Nurses
    b. The American Nurses' Association   ANA
    c. The National League for Nursing
    d. The National Association for Practical Nursing

12. Attendance at a workshop that discusses food fads and myths best illustrates an example of:
    a. Lifetime commitment
    b. Required education
    c. Nursing accountability
    d. Continuing education

SHORT ANSWER QUESTIONS

Directions: Read each of the following statements and supply the word(s) necessary in the space provided.

1. The Union government appointed Dorothea Dix, a social worker, to select and organize women volunteers to care for its Civil War troops. List four of the criteria used to select these applicants.
   a. _35 yrs - ro_____
   b. _____
   c. _____
   d. _____

2. Describe five of the rationales for acquiring continuing education.
   a. _____
   b. _____
   c. _____
   d. _____
   e. _____

3. List five of the factors affecting the choice of nursing educational programs.
   a. _____
   b. _____
   c. _____
   d. _____
   e. _____

4. List the three factors that delayed the decision to make baccalaureate education the entry level into nursing practice.
   a. _____
   b. _____
   c. _____

5. Compare the level of responsibility among practical/vocational, associate degree, and baccalaureate degree nurses for each step of the nursing process:
   _____
   _____

CRITICAL THINKING EXERCISES

1. Explain the factors that influenced your decision to choose the nursing program in which you are enrolled.

2. Describe the philosophy of your nursing program.

3. Based on your school's philosophy, construct a working model of nursing.

CHAPTER 2

Nursing Process

SUMMARY

As nursing practice takes on a more independent role, nurses are being held responsible and accountable for providing appropriate nursing interventions that reflect current acceptable standards for nursing practice.

This chapter discusses the five parts of the nursing process: assessment, nursing diagnosis, planning, implementation, and evaluation. Simply stated, assessment is gathering the appropriate and accurate data. Nursing diagnosis is the problem statement derived from accurate analysis of the data. The problem identified may be actual, possible, or potential. Planning involves putting the needs in order of priority, setting short- and long-term goals, and identifying possible options. Implementation is actually carrying out the nursing orders. Evaluation determines how effective the nursing interventions were and the degree to which each goal was met. Evaluation is an ongoing part of the nursing process and may indicate a need to revise the plan of care. When nursing practice reflects the nursing process, patients receive quality care in minimal time with maximum efficiency.

MATCHING QUESTIONS

Directions: Match the steps of the problem-solving process in Part B with the steps of the nursing process in Part A.

Part A
1. _____ Assessment
2. _____ Nursing diagnosis
3. _____ Planning
4. _____ Implementation
5. _____ Evaluation

Part B
a. The identification of desired outcomes
b. The review of the entire process
c. The collection of information
d. Carrying out the plan
e. The exact nature of the problem is identified

Directions: Match the terms in Part B with the signs and symptoms in Part A. Each of the terms in Part B *must* be used more than once.

Part A
1. _____ Pulse 140 beats/minute
2. _____ Cloudy urine
3. _____ Burns with urination
4. _____ Feeling warm
5. _____ Emesis—green liquid
6. _____ Pain in left groin

Part B
a. Subjective
b. Objective

TRUE/FALSE QUESTIONS

Directions: For items 1 through 10, decide if the statement is true or false and mark T or F in the space provided.

1. _____ Assessment data should be gathered only from the patient's record.
2. _____ A nursing diagnosis closely resembles a medical diagnosis.
3. _____ The North American Nursing Diagnosis Association uses the word *potential* when making a nursing diagnosis about a problem for which the patient is at risk.
4. _____ When setting priorities for the patient's problems, the nurse should always list them according to the hierarchy of needs.
5. _____ The terms *goals* and *outcomes* may be used synonymously.

5

6. _____ A limited collection of a few, specific related facts is known as a focus assessment.

7. _____ Validation is the process of measuring how well a goal is reached.

8. _____ A potential health problem that would require the cooperative care of the nurse and the physician is known as a collaborative problem.

9. _____ Objective data is information that only the patient can describe.

10. _____ The nursing process is within the legal scope of nursing practice.

MULTIPLE CHOICE QUESTIONS

Directions: For items 1 through 15, circle the letter that corresponds to the *best* answer for each question.

1. A change in the practice of nursing as it is today was brought about by:
   a. Nurses now directing patient care more dependably
   b. The development and use of the nursing process for providing appropriate care according to priorities of need
   c. Nurses being held accountable and responsible for providing appropriate care according to accepted standards
   d. The knowledge that nurses should continue to work interdependently with other health care professionals

2. The primary goal of the nursing process is:
   a. To set into action the process of obtaining objectives
   b. To facilitate a united effort between the patient and the nursing team to achieve the desired outcome
   c. To learn to use the steps so that nursing will be organized and more efficient
   d. To give patient care within a minimum amount of time with maximum efficiency

3. Subjective data is *best* described as:
   a. Information that is measurable and observable
   b. Information that only the patient describes
   c. Information that is lengthy and comprehensive
   d. Information that is detailed and specific

4. The step in the nursing process involved with problem identification is:
   a. Assessment
   b. Planning
   c. Diagnosis
   d. Implementation

5. Which of the following *best* supports the concept that the nursing process is dynamic:
   a. Each patient is the unique product of physical, emotional, social, and spiritual components
   b. The health status of any patient is constantly changing; the nursing process acts like a continuous loop
   c. It is important that the patient and the nurse understand the final expected outcomes and work together
   d. The nurse practice acts are expanding to describe nursing in terms of more independent roles

6. Which of the following *best* supports the concept that the nursing process is patient centered:
   a. The nursing process facilitates a plan of care for each patient as a unique individual
   b. The health status of a patient changes constantly, and one problem is often related to another
   c. It is important that the patient and nurse work together toward the expected outcome
   d. All patients have needs that must be met in order of priority, as directed by the hierarchy

7. The *best* definition of assessment is:
   a. The process of measuring how well a goal or objective is reached
   b. An expected outcome or desired end result toward which the nurse works
   c. The action of collecting and organizing patient information
   d. The acquisition of skills required to meet the needs of the patient

8. Certain physiologic problems that nurses monitor to detect onset or change in status but are beyond the scope of independent nursing practice are referred to as:
   a. Actual problems
   b. Collaborative problems
   c. Potential problems
   d. Possible problems

9. Which of the following indicate the three parts of a nursing diagnostic statement:
   a. Problem, etiology, and signs and symptoms
   b. Risk, dysfunction, and impairment
   c. Possibility, problem, and purpose
   d. Physiology, etiology, and collaboration

10. The etiology named in the nursing diagnosis is:
    a. The problem according to the patient
    b. The cause of the problem
    c. The information relating to the problem
    d. The physician's diagnosis

11. The most commonly used method for determining priorities is:
    a. For the nurse to think in terms of the hierarchy of needs
    b. For the nurse to evaluate which problems can be solved or reduced in a short time
    c. For the nurse to analyze which problem, if changed, would result in change in others
    d. For the nurse to consult with the patient concerning his wishes

12. The *best* example of a goal statement is:
    a. Mr. J. would like to walk ten steps without assistance today
    b. Mrs. B. will be discharged in a wheelchair on Sunday afternoon
    c. Mrs. S. would like to have family visitors in the evening
    d. Johnny will walk to the playroom unassisted by May 5

13. The *best* example of a nursing order is:
    a. Give 2 ounces of clear fluids every 2 hours until 10 P.M.
    b. Give clear fluids of choice when awake until 10 P.M.
    c. Change the patient's position and give him a backrub frequently
    d. Encourage the patient to breathe deeply and cough to bring up sputum

14. In terms of the nursing process, evaluation provides:
    a. Information on the degree to which the nursing assessment was correct
    b. Information on the degree to which the nursing diagnosis was correct
    c. Information on the degree to which a goal is being met through the use of specific nursing measures
    d. Information on the degree to which the patient has agreed with the plan of nursing care to be given

15. Which of the following is carried out when the results of the nursing evaluation show that the goal has not been met:
    a. The plan of care is discarded and a new plan is written
    b. The nursing orders to accomplish the goal are discontinued
    c. The nursing orders described in the plan are continued

SHORT ANSWER QUESTION

Directions: Read the following nursing diagnosis:
Impaired skin integrity related to immobility.

1. Write the words below that pertain to the etiology.
   _____

2. Write the words below that pertain to the problem.
   _____

CRITICAL THINKING EXERCISES

1. Assessment is composed of data from many sources. List four sources of data. State several examples of data you might collect from each source. Decide whether the data is subjective or objective. Explain your choices.

2. Read the short case study that follows. Underline the cues that represent a data cluster implying a nursing diagnosis. Write the diagnosis first as a two-part statement. Expand your diagnosis to a three-part statement. Ask your instructor to review and evaluate your work.

   Mrs. S., aged 93, has lived alone since the death of her husband 20 years ago. Until recently she has been able to manage her own self-care and medications. Her son and his family live next door and provide her with transportation and socialization.

   About four months ago, Mrs. S. decided she could no longer get out of bed. She began forgetting to eat, bathe, and take her medications. Her short-term memory began to fail and she lost track of time. She now spends approximately 20 hours per day in bed. She requires assistance to get up, walks with a walker, and her son and his wife must bring her meals to her and administer her medications. Several times a day she says, "I'm worried about what will become of me. I'm too old. I feel so helpless. I want to go to a rest home."

   Two months later, she is a resident in a nursing home. She gets up to a chair with assistance, is incontinent of bowel and bladder, and is unable to swallow. Most of the time she is not aware of time or place.

CHAPTER 3

Laws and Ethics

SUMMARY

In the United States, laws are designed to empower federal, state, and local governments to ensure the health and safety of citizens, protect the public welfare, and uphold individual rights and freedom. In this chapter, the student will find a brief overview of laws as they apply to nursing. Common crimes and torts, as well as laws that affect nursing practices are discussed. The role of the state board of nursing as the regulatory agency for managing the education, licensure, and clinical practice of nurses in the state is briefly described.

MATCHING QUESTIONS

Directions: For items 1 through 6, match the definitions in Part B with the terms in Part A.

Part A
1. _____ Libel
2. _____ Assault
3. _____ Lawsuit
4. _____ Battery
5. _____ Slander
6. _____ Malpractice

Part B
a. An untruthful oral statement about a person that subjects him to ridicule or contempt
b. A threat or an attempt to make bodily contact with another person without the person's consent
c. Alleged professional negligence
d. An untruthful written statement about a person that subjects her to ridicule or contempt
e. A wrong committed by a person against another person or his property
f. A legal action in a court
g. A wrong committed against persons or property (the act is considered to be against the public)
h. Bodily contact with another person without the person's consent

Directions: For items 7 through 12, match the descriptions in Part B with the types of law in Part A.

Part A
7. _____ Administrative laws
8. _____ Nurse practice acts
9. _____ Criminal laws
10. _____ Civil laws
11. _____ Statutes of limitation
12. _____ Laws

Part B
a. Rules of conduct
b. Protect personal rights and freedom
c. Protect the public's welfare
d. Establish a time frame for litigation
e. Give state and federal governments legal authority
f. Define the unique role of the nurse

MULTIPLE CHOICE QUESTIONS

Directions: For items 1 through 10, circle the letter that corresponds to the best answer for each question.

1. A tort is defined as:
   a. A legal action involving an act or its omission that harms someone
   b. An untruthful written statement about a person that subjects him to ridicule or contempt
   c. A threat or an attempt to make bodily contact with another person without the person's consent
   d. An illegal act that violates the right of a person to avoid public attention

2. The most used and distributed copies of the "Patient's Bill of Rights" was prepared by:
   a. The American Nurses' Association
   b. The American Medical Association
   c. The Federation of Licensed Practical Nurses
   d. The American Hospital Association

9

3. An incident report is best described as:
   a. A personal written account of an event
   b. A written account of an unusual event that may cause harm
   c. A contract between a person and a company willing to provide legal service
   d. A lawsuit alleging a professional's failure to act responsibly caused harm

4. A situation that results in an injury although the person did not intend to cause harm is called:
   a. Negligence
   b. False imprisonment
   c. Defamation
   d. Unintentional tort

5. Which of the following is true regarding Good Samaritan laws:
   a. They provide nurses with absolute exemption from prosecution
   b. They establish a designated amount within which a lawsuit can be filed
   c. They provide legal immunity for persons who give first aid at the scene of an accident

6. Ethics is best defined as:
   a. A list of written statements describing ideal behavior for members of a particular group
   b. A rule of conduct established and enforced by the government of a society
   c. Laws passed by each state that protect the public from persons considered unfit to practice nursing
   d. A system of moral or philosophical principles that directs actions as being either right or wrong

7. Which of the following best defines code of ethics:
   a. A system of moral or philosophical principles that directs actions as being either right or wrong
   b. A system identifying the rights of individuals and respecting those rights
   c. A list of rights that arise from social customs and religious traditions
   d. A list of written statements describing ideal behavior for a group of individuals

8. The nurse practice acts are identified and published by:
   a. The state legislatures
   b. The federal government
   c. The National League for Nursing
   d. The American Nurses' Association

9. Of the following statements, which best relates to the characteristic that nursing practice is self-regulated:
   a. Most states appoint nurses to boards that evaluate nursing educational programs
   b. Nurses now hold membership in various organizations that are dedicated to improving the quality of nursing practice
   c. Because nursing is a lifetime commitment, nurses are devoting more interest and energy to its advancement
   d. Nursing practice has evolved from a historically dependent role to one that has increasing independence

10. Which statement *best* describes deontology:
    a. Ethical study based on moral obligation
    b. A choice between two undesirable outcomes
    c. Proposal that all patients be told the truth
    d. Ethical theory based on final outcome

TRUE OR FALSE QUESTIONS

Directions: For items 1 through 10, decide if the statement is true or false and mark T or F in the space provided.

1. _____ The law that gives certain persons legal protection when they give aid to someone in an emergency is referred to as the Good Samaritan law.

2. _____ Invasion of privacy is unjustifiable restraint or prevention of the movement of a person without proper consent.

3. _____ The prolongation of life with various types of equipment may cause the nurse to face an ethical dilemma.

4. _____ According to the "Patient's Bill of Rights," an individual has the right to refuse treatment.

5. _____ The advice "follow your conscience" is one of the guidelines given for dealing with ethical decisions.

6. _____ The nurse is responsible for giving the patient information concerning his medical treatment as prescribed by the physician.

7. _____ Advanced directives are considered legal in all 50 states.

8. _____ There are nurse practice acts in all 50 states, but the laws vary considerably.

9. _____ The person accused of breaking the law is called the plaintiff.

10. _____ Even though health agencies carry liability insurance, it is suggested that student and graduate nurses carry their own insurance also.

SHORT ANSWER QUESTIONS

Directions: Read each of the following statements and supply the word(s) necessary in the space provided.

1. List the four elements that must be proven in a negligence or malpractice case.

   a. _____

   b. _____

   c. _____

   d. _____

2. List five common ethical issues that nurses encounter in everyday practice.

   a. _____

   b. _____

   c. _____

   d. _____

   e. _____

CRITICAL THINKING EXERCISES

1. A client with end stage renal disease says she wants to die and asks for assistance. Describe how two nurses with differing ideas of what is morally right and wrong might respond.

2. Explain how a professional code of ethics differs from a personal sense of what is morally right and wrong.

3. Interview a nurse who is a member of a hospital ethics committee. Describe the nurse's role on this committee. Does it differ from the role(s) of other members of this same committee?

CHAPTER 4

Health and Illness

SUMMARY

Health is a goal to which nursing is committed. However, it is a predictable characteristic of human nature that there will be changes in health. One cannot expect to stay healthy forever. In this context, nurses are committed to helping individuals prevent illness and restore or improve their health.

In this discussion, health is defined recognizing individual differences and values. Spiritual, emotional, social, and physical well being is described within the scope of the individual's rights and obligations for health promotion and maintenance. Most Americans believe that health is a resource, a right and a personal responsibility. Because of its dynamic state, health is depicted as a continuum from high-level wellness to death. The individual functions within a wide range of variations at any given time. The concept of a hierarchy of human needs that motivate behavior is introduced. Nurses use this hierarchy to assist in identifying the area of priority requiring nursing intervention. The needs on the lowest tier must be met first.

MATCHING QUESTIONS

Directions: For items 1 through 12, match Maslow's Hierarchy of Needs in Part B with the human needs in Part A. (Note: The choices in Part B may be used more than once.)

Part A
1. _____ Love
2. _____ Rest
3. _____ Safety
4. _____ Protection
5. _____ Esteem
6. _____ Exploration
7. _____ Food
8. _____ Closeness
9. _____ Sex
10. _____ Air
11. _____ Activity
12. _____ Water

Part B
a. Physiologic
b. Safety and security
c. Love and belonging
d. Self-esteem
e. Self-actualization

MULTIPLE CHOICE QUESTIONS

Directions: For items 1 through 12, circle the letter that corresponds to the best answer for each question.

1. The term health is best described as:
   a. A generally accepted right belonging to everyone
   b. An acceptable quality of life as defined by the individual who is experiencing the problem
   c. A state of complete physical, mental, and social well-being and not merely the absence of disease
   d. A state of being which cannot always be maintained and acquired alone

2. The term morbidity refers to:
   a. The incidence of a specific disease
   b. The number of deaths per unit of population
   c. A state of discomfort due to impaired health
   d. The disappearance of signs and symptoms

3. Which of the following are true concerning the state of wellness:
   a. A state in which body organs function normally
   b. A state in which one feels safe
   c. A state of discomfort in which one's health is impaired as a result of injury, stress, disease or an accident
   d. A state in which one feels a balanced integration of physical, emotional, social, and spiritual health

13

4. Which of the following statements best describes acute illness:
   a. One that comes on slowly and lasts a long time
   b. One in which there is no potential for cure
   c. One that comes on suddenly and is of short duration
   d. One that has developed independently of other disease

5. An idiopathic illness is best described as:
   a. One that is acquired from the parents' genetic codes
   b. One that is present at birth
   c. One for which there is no known cause
   d. One that results from permanent organ damage

6. The method of nursing care in which each nurse on a patient unit is assigned specific tasks is known as:
   a. Primary nursing
   b. Functional nursing
   c. Team nursing
   d. Nurse-managed care

7. Providing nursing care by the case method involves:
   a. Assigning specific tasks to each nurse on the patient unit
   b. Assigning one nurse to administer all the care a patient needs for the shift
   c. Assigning one nurse the responsibility of the patient's 24-hour care
   d. Assigning many nursing personnel to care for a group of patients until all the work is complete

8. Of the following, which best describes the concept of team nursing:
   a. The patient's total 24-hour care is the responsibility of one nurse
   b. Each of the nurses on a patient unit is assigned a specific task
   c. Many nursing personnel divide the patient care and all work until it is completed
   d. The head nurse plans the patient care and then all of the nurses work until it is completed

9. The nursing care that is similar to the principles practiced by a successful business is:
   a. Primary nursing
   b. Nurse-managed care
   c. Team nursing
   d. Functional nursing

10. The term continuity of care refers to:
    a. A continuum of health care
    b. A method of providing care
    c. A network of health care services
    d. A group of health care specialists

TRUE OR FALSE QUESTIONS

Directions: For items I through 10, decide if the statement is true or false and mark T or F in the space provided.

1. _____ A chronic illness is one that comes on slowly and lasts a relatively short time.
2. _____ Functional nursing is one of the most-practiced methods of nursing.
3. _____ Health is a state in which the body organs function normally.
4. _____ Remission is the term used to describe the period during an illness when the symptoms subside.
5. _____ Wellness is more than just the absence of physical symptoms.
6. _____ A state in which one feels safe, well liked, and productive is known as spiritual well being.
7. _____ The primary nurse is accountable for the patient's care even though he or she may be off duty.
8. _____ Health could be measured by the patient's physical, emotional, social, and spiritual well being.
9. _____ Because health is an intangible substance, it is not considered a resource.
10. _____ Functional nursing tends to focus more on the tasks to be completed than on the patient's needs.

CRITICAL THINKING EXERCISES

Research each of the following methods of administering patient care, and do the following:

   Primary Nursing
   Team Nursing
   Functional Nursing
   Nurse-Managed Care

   a. List the characteristics of the method
   b. Identify the individual who is responsible and accountable
   c. State one advantage and one disadvantage of the method
   d. Give an example of the type of health care facility in which this method could be used

CHAPTER 5

Homeostasis, Adaptation, and Stress

SUMMARY

Health is a tenuous state. To sustain it, the body continuously adapts to changes that have the potential for disturbing equilibrium. As long as the stressors are minor, the response is negligible, occurring quite unnoticed. However, when a stressor is intense or when multiple stressors occur at the same time, the effort to restore balance may result in uncomfortable signs and symptoms many call "stress." If stress is prolonged, stress-related disorders and even death may occur. This chapter explores the nature of homeostasis, adaptive mechanisms for homeostatic regulation, the effect of stress, and nursing interventions that promote and restore health.

MATCHING QUESTIONS

Directions: For items 1 through 6, match the descriptions given in Part B with the terms in Part A.

Part A

1. _____ Holism
2. _____ Stress
3. _____ Adaptation
4. _____ Coping mechanism
5. _____ Homeostasis
6. _____ Stress management

Part B

a. Therapeutic activities used to reestablish physiologic balance
b. A stable state of physiologic equilibrium
c. Manner in which an organism responds to change
d. Implies multiple entities contributing to the whole person
e. Unconscious tactics used to protect the psyche
f. Describes reactions that occur when equilibrium is disturbed

Directions: For items 7 through 12, match the categories given in Part B with the stressors in Part A. (Note: Each answer may be used more than once.)

Part A

7. _____ Guilt
8. _____ Gender
9. _____ Aging
10. _____ Hopelessness
11. _____ Bitterness
12. _____ Poverty

Part B

a. Physiologic
b. Psychologic
c. Social
d. Spiritual

Directions: For items 13 through 20, match the examples given in Part B with the coping mechanisms in Part A.

Part A

13. _____ Suppression
14. _____ Rationalization
15. _____ Somatization
16. _____ Reaction formation
17. _____ Identification
18. _____ Displacement
19. _____ Denial
20. _____ Sublimation

Part B

a. Developing diarrhea to stay home from work
b. Imitating the way your boss dresses and talks
c. "Sleeping on the problem"
d. Becoming a sports announcer when you can't be an athlete
e. Kicking the wastebasket after your boss reprimands you
f. Blaming failure on a test on how it was constructed
g. Being extremely nice to someone you really dislike
h. Refusing to believe your best friend has terminal cancer

15

MULTIPLE CHOICE QUESTIONS

Directions: For items 1 through 10, circle the letter that corresponds to the best answer for each question.

1. The term homeostasis refers to:
   a. Negligible responses that come about unnoticed
   b. The relationship between the mind and the body
   c. A relatively stable state of physiologic equilibrium
   d. A philosophic concept of interrelatedness in humans

2. The autonomic nervous system is composed of:
   a. The reticular activating system near the cortex
   b. Peripheral nerves that affect physiologic function
   c. The structures in the midbrain and the brain stem
   d. A collective group of glands located throughout the body

3. The function of the parasympathetic nervous system is to:
   a. Accelerate physiologic functions necessary for "fight or flight"
   b. Regulate and maintain physiologic activities that promote survival
   c. Allow for abstract thought, use of language, and decision making
   d. Inhibit physiologic stimulation resulting from "fight or flight"

4. Behaving in a manner that is characteristic of a younger age best describes which of the following coping mechanisms?
   a. Displacement
   b. Regression
   c. Rationalization
   d. Repression

5. The general adaptation syndrome refers to:
   a. The collective physiologic processes that take place in response to a stressor
   b. The collection of diseases and disorders that result from prolonged exposure to stress
   c. The collection of techniques available to promote physiologic comfort and well-being
   d. The collection of potential stressors that particularly affect patients in the hospital

6. The Social Readjustment Rating Scale was developed by:
   a. Holmes and Watson
   b. Abraham Maslow
   c. Dorothea Orem
   d. Holmes and Rahe

7. Powerlessness is an example of which of the following categories of stressors:
   a. Physiologic
   b. Psychologic
   c. Social
   d. Spiritual

8. Rapid heart rate, rapid breathing, and dry mouth are examples of which of the following categories of signs and symptoms of stress:
   a. Physical
   b. Emotional
   c. Cognitive
   d. Affective

TRUE OR FALSE QUESTIONS

Directions: For items 1 through 10, decide if the statement is true or false and mark T or F in the space provided.

1. _____ When internal or external changes overwhelm homeostatic adaptation, stress results.
2. _____ Forgetfulness is a physical sign of increased stress.
3. _____ Coping mechanisms enable individuals to maintain their mental equilibrium.
4. _____ The general adaptation syndrome describes the pathologic effects of the overuse of stress reduction techniques.
5. _____ Responses to stress may be mediated by interactions that manipulate sensory stimuli.
6. _____ An individual's attitudes and values may affect his response to stressors.
7. _____ Irritability, withdrawal, and depression are common physical signs and symptoms of increased stress.
8. _____ Gastritis and irritable bowel syndrome are examples of stress-related disorders.
9. _____ Bruxism is a synonym for snoring.
10. _____ Accusing a person of a race different from your own of being prejudiced is an example of regression.

CRITICAL THINKING EXERCISE

Investigate one stress management technique that is available in your area. Prepare a brief report that includes:

    a. time required to learn and use the activity

    b. the cost

    c. how many complete the program

    d. the target population

Include an analysis of the effectiveness of the technique.

Culture and Ethnicity

SUMMARY

No two patients are ever exactly alike. Nurses have always cared for patients with various kinds of differences. These variations include, but are not limited to, age, gender, race, health status, religion, education, occupation, and income. Culture and ethnicity, the focus of this chapter, are yet other ways patients may vary. Despite the existence of these characteristics, the tendency has been to treat all patients alike. This type of care, acultural nursing, may be politically popular but it may not be in the best interest of promoting, maintaining, or restoring health.

The time has come to promote "transcultural nursing," a term conceived in the 1970s to describe nursing within the context of another's culture. This kind of nursing care requires acceptance of each patient as an individual, knowledge of health problems that affect particular cultural groups, planning of health care within the patient's belief system, and respect for alternative health practices.

MATCHING QUESTIONS

Directions: For items 1 through 5, match the definitions in Part B with the terms in Part A.

Part A

1. _____ Culture
2. _____ Race
3. _____ Ethnicity
4. _____ Stereotype
5. _____ Subculture

Part B

a. A unique cultural group that coexists with a dominant group
b. Values, beliefs, and practices of a particular group
c. A fixed attitude toward a particular group
d. Refers to biologic variations
e. Bond of kinship with a country

Directions: For items 6 through 10, match the corresponding health beliefs in Part B with the subcultures in Part A.

Part A

6. _____ Anglo American
7. _____ African American
8. _____ Asian American
9. _____ Latino
10. _____ Native American

Part B

a. Illness results when equilibrium is disturbed.
b. Illness occurs when Mother Earth is disturbed.
c. Illness is caused by microorganisms.
d. Illness occurs as a punishment from God.
e. Illness is caused by supernatural forces.

MULTIPLE CHOICE QUESTIONS

Directions: For items 1 through 9, circle the letter that corresponds to the best answer for each question.

1. The term transcultural nursing refers to:
   a. The confusion one experiences when exposed to culturally atypical behavior
   b. The ability to provide care within the context of another's culture and beliefs
   c. The ability to speak a second language as part of one's culture
   d. The belief that one's own ethnicity is superior to all others

2. Of the 270 tribes of Native Americans present in the United States today, which of the following is the largest:
    a. The Navajos
    b. The Sioux
    c. The Eskimos
    d. The Aleuts

3. There are several drugs that may precipitate the anemic response G-6-PD in African Americans. From the list below, select the name of one of these drugs:
    a. Calcium
    b. Probenecid
    c. Acetic acid
    d. Lactase

4. The drug referred to in question 3 is used to treat which of the following health problems:
    a. Malaria
    b. Urinary infections
    c. Gout
    d. Respiratory infections

5. A lactase deficiency is exhibited as intolerance for which of the following products:
    a. Dairy products
    b. Alcohol
    c. Artificial sweeteners
    d. Kosher foods

6. From the following, choose the phrases that are true regarding the way(s) in which an individual demonstrates pride in one's ethnicity:
    a. Placing value on specific physical characteristics
    b. Giving one's children ethnic names
    c. Wearing special items of clothing
    d. All of the above are true statements

7. Which of the following represent four leading causes of death across all subcultures in the United States:
    a. HIV infection, diabetes, cancer, suicide
    b. Pneumonia, diabetes, heart disease, suicide
    c. Heart disease, cancer, stroke, injuries
    d. Influenza, pneumonia, stroke, injuries

8. The belief that illness occurs when the harmony of nature is disturbed is common among which of the following U.S. subcultures:
    a. Native Americans
    b. Latinos
    c. African Americans
    d. Asian Americans

9. Those methods of disease treatment or prevention that are outside conventional practices are called:
    a. Castigo de Dios
    b. Yin and yang
    c. Shaman
    d. Folk medicine

TRUE OR FALSE QUESTIONS

Directions: For items 1 through 10, decide if the statement is true or false and mark T or F in the space provided.

1. _____ It is appropriate to assume that everyone who affiliates with a particular group behaves exactly alike.

2. _____ Cultural attitudes are learned by example and are passed on from one generation to the next.

3. _____ Eskimos and Aleuts are included among the Native American tribes of North America.

4. _____ Daily bathing, use of deodorant, and shaving are standard hygiene practices in the Anglo American culture.

5. _____ Acupuncture, acupressure, and herbs are used by many Asian Americans to restore health and balance.

6. _____ If a translator is required, choose one who is male and older than the patient to be certain the patient feels secure.

7. _____ If a patient of a subculture different from the nurse's appears confused by a question, the nurse should repeat the question using simple words and shorter sentences.

8. _____ As a whole, Americans are time oriented and schedule their activities according to clock hours.

9. _____ Prayer and penance, spiritual healers, and eating foods that are "hot" or "cold" are common health practices among Asian Americans.

10. _____ Facilitating rituals by whomever the client identifies as a healer within his or her belief system is a means of demonstrating culturally sensitive nursing care.

SHORT ANSWER QUESTIONS

Directions: Read each of the following statements and supply the word(s) necessary in the space provided.

1. List five characteristics of Anglo American culture.
   a. _____
   b. _____
   c. _____
   d. _____
   e. _____

2. As discussed in the text, list three ways of demonstrating cultural sensitivity.
   a. _____
   b. _____
   c. _____

CRITICAL THINKING EXERCISES

1. A new post partum Samoan woman is wearing a large kerchief around her abdomen. Discuss how it would be best to inquire about this practice from a culturally sensitive perspective.

2. Discuss how an Anglo-American nurse and her Asian-American patient might experience culture shock during a health care encounter.

3. Research ways your community is culturally diverse. How are the health care needs of the population being met? How can health care be improved?

CHAPTER 7

The Nurse–Patient Relationship

SUMMARY

Nurses provide services, or skills, that assist individuals, called patients or clients, to resolve health problems that are beyond their own capabilities or to cope with those that will not improve. There are several differences between the services that nurses provide and those provided by other caring people.

An intangible factor that helps place nurses in high regard is the relationship that develops between nurses and patients. One of the primary keys to establishing and maintaining a positive nurse–patient relationship is the manner and style of a nurse's communication.

MATCHING QUESTIONS

Directions: For items 1 through 6, match the examples in Part B with the communication techniques in Part A.

Part A
1. _____ Informing
2. _____ Open-ended questioning
3. _____ Reflecting
4. _____ Clarifying
5. _____ Confronting
6. _____ Summarizing

Part B
a. Patient: "I'm miserable." Nurse: "Miserable?"
b. "You want to go home but you haven't been doing your exercises."
c. "Are you having any pain?"
d. "How does your pain feel?"
e. "We've talked about health and exercise. Would you like to join a health club?"
f. "Your physician will be in at 9:30 this morning."
g. Patient: "I can't deal with it anymore." Nurse: "Tell me what it is that you are unable to deal with."

Directions: For items 7 through 12, match the examples in Part B with the nontherapeutic communication techniques in Part A.

Part A
7. _____ False reassurance
8. _____ Clichés
9. _____ Belittling
10. _____ Patronizing
11. _____ Disagreeing
12. _____ Approval

Part B
a. Nurse: "I'm glad you're exercising so regularly."
b. Nurse: "Are we ready to take our medicine now?"
c. Nurse: "Where did you get an idea like that?"
d. Nurse: "You can do it, you're a tough old bird."
e. Nurse: "Lots of people learn to do this."
f. Nurse: "Everything will be just fine."

MULTIPLE CHOICE QUESTIONS

Directions: For items 1 through 10, circle the letter that corresponds to the best answer for each question.

1. The example that best relates to the concept that nurses promote independence is:
   a. The nurse gives Miss H. a syringe, a needle, and an orange and tells her to practice injections
   b. The nurse selects the appropriate foods from Miss H.'s menu for her diabetic diet
   c. The nurse uses communication skills to assist Miss H. with her fears about diabetes
   d. The nurse demonstrates to Miss H. the procedures for preparing an insulin injection

2. When developing a therapeutic nurse–patient relationship, a desired outcome is:
   a. Developing a friendship
   b. Making the patient comfortable
   c. Moving toward restoring health
   d. Learning to know oneself

3. Of the following situations, which relates to the introductory phase of the nurse–patient relationship:
   a. The nurse uses communication skills to learn about Mr. J.'s health problems during the admission procedure
   b. The nurse explains to Mr. J. that he will have to assist with some of his care while he is in the hospital
   c. The nurse shares her information about Mr. J. with the other nursing personnel that will be caring for him
   d. The nurse plans and follows through with discharge teaching when it is time for Mr. J. to go home

4. An example of verbal communication is:
   a. Moaning
   b. Laughing
   c. Writing
   d. Crying

5. An example of nonverbal communication is:
   a. Speaking
   b. Moaning
   c. Reading
   d. Writing

6. An obstacle to effective communication would be:
   a. Using the principles of touch by giving the patient a backrub
   b. Accepting what the patient says while being alert to what he is not saying
   c. Asking the patient if she feels lonely or sad
   d. Interrupting the patient when he seems to be deep in thought

7. When the nurse stops in during the evening, Mrs. D. states that she is very worried about her operation tomorrow. Of the following responses, which would be the most appropriate:
   a. "That is very understandable, Mrs. D., would you like to talk about your operation?"
   b. "Don't worry—everything is going to be okay."
   c. "That's just a routine operation that you are having. No need to worry about it."
   d. "You'll be okay—your doctor and our operating room staff do these procedures every day"

8. The term kinesics refers to:
   a. Vocal sounds that are not actually words
   b. The use of space to communicate
   c. The use of body language to communicate
   d. The use of tactile stimuli to communicate

9. Which of the following statements best describes task-oriented touch:
   a. The personal contact required to perform nursing procedures
   b. The personal contact used to demonstrate concern for another
   c. The personal contact required to maintain safety for older adults
   d. The personal contact used to demonstrate affection for another

10. It is suggested that the nurse sit in a relaxed position at eye level with the patient when communicating with a patient because:
    a. This indicates that the nurse is fully involved in what is being communicated
    b. If the patient feels rushed, he may interpret this to be disinterest by the nurse
    c. Responses to stress are manifested through active listening on the part of the nurse
    d. People have less control over nonverbal communication than they do over verbal communication

TRUE OR FALSE QUESTIONS

Directions: For items 1 through 10, decide if the statement is true or false and mark T or F in the space provided.

1. _____ Intimate space is reserved for sharing conversations that are not intended to be private.

2. _____ One of the most important nursing skills is the promotion of the patient's independent ability to meet her own health needs.

3. _____ It is okay to use the titles "gramps" or "granny" to develop a therapeutic relationship with an elderly patient.

4. _____ Nursing acts are prompted by observing an individual in distress.

5. _____ Identifying the problem, describing desired outcomes, and answering questions honestly are nursing responsibilities within the nurse–patient relationship.

6. _____ For older adults, touching may be more important than talking.

7. _____ A therapeutic nurse–patient relationship is more likely to develop when the nurse accepts that the patient has the potential for growth and change.

8. _____ The introductory phase of the nurse–patient relationship involves mutually planning the patient's care.

9. _____ No relationship can exist without verbal and nonverbal communication.

10. _____ Therapeutic communication refers to using words and gestures to accomplish an objective.

SHORT ANSWER QUESTIONS

Directions: Read each of the following statements and supply the word(s) necessary in the space provided.

1. List three therapeutic uses of silence.
   a. _____
   b. _____
   c. _____

2. List the principles that provide the basis for a therapeutic nurse–patient relationship.
   a. _____
   b. _____
   c. _____
   d. _____
   e. _____

3. Explain the difference between task-related touch and affective touch.
   _____
   _____

CRITICAL THINKING EXERCISES

1. Work with another student and attempt to express each of the following without using verbal communication:
   a. pain
   b. fear of discomfort
   c. an uncaring attitude
   d. genuine concern for your client

2. Describe communication techniques that the nurse might use to communicate with an unconscious client in a critical care unit.

3. Discuss principles of communication appropriate to older adults.

CHAPTER 8

Patient Teaching

SUMMARY

One of the many means by which nurses apply communication skills is through the role of teacher. Health teaching promotes the patient's independent ability to meet his or her own health needs. As patient advocates, nurses help clients use health information to make informed decisions about their health care. Health teaching is no longer an optional nursing activity; many state nurse practice acts require it. Client teaching is a requirement of acceptable nursing care according to ANA Standards of Nursing Practice. Patient records must show what has been taught and present evidence that learning did indeed take place. Limited hospitalization demands that health teaching begin as soon after admission as possible.

MATCHING QUESTIONS

Directions: For items 1 through 17, match the categories of the learner in Part B with the characteristics in Part A. (Note: Categories may be used more than once.)

Part A
1. _____ Compulsory learner
2. _____ Active leaner
3. _____ Needs structure
4. _____ Motivated by own interest
5. _____ Learning is problem-centered
6. _____ Short attention span
7. _____ Practical thinker
8. _____ Motivated by need
9. _____ Rote learner
10. _____ Goal oriented
11. _____ Concrete thinker
12. _____ Needs frequent feedback
13. _____ Responds to family encouragement
14. _____ Task oriented
15. _____ Passive
16. _____ Subject centered
17. _____ Crisis learner

Part B
a. Pedagogic learner
b. Androgogic learner
c. Gerogogic learner

Directions: For items 18 through 27, match the domains in Part B with the behaviors in Part A. (Note: The domains may be used more than once.)

Part A
18. _____ Remove
19. _____ Promote
20. _____ List
21. _____ Empty
22. _____ Locate
23. _____ Identify
24. _____ Assemble
25. _____ Advocate
26. _____ Change
27. _____ Label

Part B
a. Cognitive domain
b. Psychomotor domain
c. Affective domain

MULTIPLE CHOICE QUESTIONS

Directions: For items 1 through 15, circle the letter that corresponds to the best answer for each question.

1. An example of cognitive learning is:
   a. A demonstration of correct injection technique
   b. Successful completion of a test about anatomy
   c. Understanding one's anger over having cancer
   d. Expressing excitement over learning to give an injection.

2. Which of the following would be an example of learning in the psychomotor domain:
   a. Reciting the alphabet
   b. Identifying leaves from various trees
   c. Refusing to talk to strangers
   d. Assembling a puzzle

3. For the visually impaired patient, it is easier to read:
   a. Large print in black ink on white paper
   b. Small print in black ink on white paper
   c. Large print in blue ink on off-white glossy paper
   d. Small print in blue ink on off-white glossy paper

4. For the hearing impaired patient, the nurse can facilitate communication by:
   a. Talking louder, using simple words, and lowering voice pitch
   b. Sitting or standing beside the patient's "bad" ear when talking
   c. Selecting words that do not begin with the letters F, S, or K
   d. Raising the voice pitch, talking softly, and repeating the words

5. When instructing an older adult, it is important to:
   a. Reduce noise and distraction
   b. Sit at eye level beside the patient
   c. Speak rapidly and distinctly
   d. Use sentences with 12 words or less

6. Which of the following statements is true of pedagogic learners:
   a. Learning is outcome oriented
   b. Learning is self-centered
   c. Learning requires structure and encouragement
   d. Learning is motivated by reward or punishment

7. The term literacy refers to:
   a. The ability to process information
   b. Below-average intellectual capacity
   c. The ability to read and write
   d. The consequences of a learning disability

8. Scheduling a return demonstration with a client who has just been taught self-injection is an example of which step of the nursing process:
   a. Assessment
   b. Planning
   c. Implementation
   d. Evaluation

9. Of the following learning activities, which is the most effective for increasing learner retention:
   a. Reading
   b. Listening
   c. Demonstrating
   d. Observing

10. Informal teaching refers to situations in which:
    a. Teaching is unplanned and spontaneous
    b. Lessons are planned and scheduled
    c. Teaching is haphazard and occurs when the patient asks
    d. Lessons have set guidelines and follow a model

11. An appropriate time for teaching the patient would be:
    a. At the time the nurse is doing the admission interview
    b. At the time the nurse is giving medication for pain
    c. When the patient needs fluids to lower his high fever
    d. When the patient is physically and psychologically ready

12. Learning a neuromuscular skill is:
    a. In the cognitive domain
    b. In the psychomotor domain
    c. In the affective domain
    d. In the neurological domain

13. Select the cognitive domain behavior from the following list:
    a. Advocate
    b. Identify
    c. Assemble
    d. Remove

14. Which of the following is an example of informal teaching:
    a. Discussing the importance of good hygiene during the patient's bath
    b. Discussing prenatal diet principles during a class for young couples
    c. Explaining hospital policies during the admission procedure
    d. Teaching only when the patient requests information

15. Optimum learning takes place when the individual has:
    a. A command of the English language
    b. A purpose for acquiring new information
    c. The desire to please others
    d. The opportunity to attend formal classes

TRUE OR FALSE QUESTIONS

Directions: For items 1 through 10, decide if the statement is true or false and mark T or F in the space provided.

1. _____ Teaching is more effective when the client is included in the planning.
2. _____ The patient's level of literacy is not difficult to assess.
3. _____ Learning objectives provide the basis for evaluating whether learning has taken place.
4. _____ Health teaching is an optional nursing activity.
5. _____ A thorough assessment of the patient and the factors affecting learning helps to identify learning needs accurately.
6. _____ Ceiling lights tend to diffuse light, making it easier for a visually impaired patient to see.
7. _____ Knowledge of the communication process is necessary for effective client teaching.
8. _____ An acceptable motivation for learning is to "avoid criticism."
9. _____ Nurse-teachers must be able to communicate effectively with individuals and small groups.
10. _____ Culture and ethnicity have no effect on how health teaching needs are met.

SHORT ANSWER QUESTIONS

Directions: Read each of the following statements and supply the word(s) necessary in the space provided.

1. List at least three characteristics that are unique to gerogogic learners.
   a. _____
   b. _____
   c. _____

2. Identify four factors that are assessed before teaching can begin.
   a. _____
   b. _____
   c. _____
   d. _____

CRITICAL THINKING EXERCISES

1. What teaching strategies from the cognitive, affective, and psychomotor domains would be required to teach a 10-year-old how to inject his own insulin? How would you alter your teaching strategies for an older adult?

2. Give examples of how to determine if the information was actually learned for each of the situations described in Question 1.

3. Refer to Questions 1 and 2. What would be appropriate documentation for the patient's record to indicate that both teaching and learning had occurred?

CHAPTER 9

Recording and Reporting

SUMMARY

When the patient requires care from health practitioners, a legal document called a patient record will be kept. Sharing information pertinent to a patient's care is an important function among health care providers. In this chapter, various methods of organizing and recording this information are presented.

MATCHING QUESTIONS

Directions: For items 1 through 10, match the meanings in Part B with the abbreviations in Part A.

Part A
1. _____ BRP
2. _____ NKA
3. _____ NPO
4. _____ OD
5. _____ OS
6. _____ PO
7. _____ WC
8. _____ s̄
9. _____ c
10. _____ DC

Part B
a. Bowel movement
b. Without
c. Left eye
d. Discontinue
e. No known allergies
f. Before noon
g. Soap suds
h. Nothing by mouth
i. Bathroom privileges
j. By mouth
k. Right eye
l. Wheelchair
m. With

MULTIPLE CHOICE QUESTIONS

Directions: For items 1 through 11, circle the letter that corresponds to the best answer for each question.

1. On the patient's record, entries are dated and written in chronological order because:
   a. They provide a permanent accounting of a patient's health care
   b. They provide a method for keeping health personnel informed
   c. They ensure safety and continuity in the patient's care
   d. They provide a method for the collection of data for research

2. Patient care information is shared in order to:
   a. Provide a permanent accounting of a patient's health care
   b. Provide a method for keeping health personnel informed
   c. Ensure safety and continuity in the patient's care
   d. Provide a method for the collection of data for research

3. Entries on the patient's record should be objective, accurate, and legible because:
   a. The patient records are used by all health personnel in the health agency
   b. The patient records are the property of the health agency and must be kept neat
   c. The patient has a right to read her chart; therefore, it must be legible and accurate
   d. The patient records are admissible as evidence in courts of law in this country

4. A characteristic of a traditional record is:
   a. It allows only physicians and nurses to enter information
   b. It is organized according to the source of the information
   c. It is organized according to the patient's specific problems
   d. It allows health care personnel to record on the same form

5. A characteristic of the problem-oriented record is:
   a. It allows only physicians and nurses to enter information
   b. It is organized according to the source of the information
   c. It is organized according to the patient's specific problems
   d. Its organization leads to fragmentation of the patient's care

6. Which of the following are the four major parts of the problem-oriented record?
   a. Database, physician's order, problem list, and progress notes
   b. Database, problem list, nurse's notes, and progress notes
   c. Physician's orders, problem list, initial plan, and progress notes
   d. Database, problem list, initial plan, and progress notes

7. A disadvantage of narrative charting is:
   a. Every member of the health care team writes entries on the same form
   b. The patient's problems may be entered once on the nursing care plan
   c. It requires the institution to develop comprehensive documents describing norms and standards
   d. It tends to produce bulky, fragmented information with each health care person writing on separate forms

8. The method of charting in which the assessments are documented on a separate form is called:
   a. SOAP charting
   b. PIE charting
   c. Narrative charting
   d. Focus charting

9. Which of the following statements best relates to the patient's right to obtain information from his records?
   a. The patient has the right to read his record at any time
   b. Each agency has a policy about patients reading their records
   c. The patient must obtain a court order to view his records
   d. The record cannot be seen without permission from the physician

10. Convert 3:30 P.M. to military time:
    a. 1530
    b. 1330
    c. 3030
    d. 0330

11. The best reason for writing or printing clearly when making an entry on a patient's record is:
    a. Illegible entries become questionable information in a court of law
    b. Errors and omissions are likely when information is gathered by many individuals
    c. The charting legibly verifies that the medical and nursing plan was carried out
    d. Correcting an error must be done so that the words first recorded can be clearly read

TRUE OR FALSE QUESTIONS

Directions: For items 1 through 12, decide if the statement is true or false and mark T or F in the space provided.

1. _____ Specific requirements on the frequency for charting vary from agency to agency.

2. _____ Entries on a patient's record should only be made by the physician and the nurses responsible for her care.

3. _____ The traditional record is organized according to a patient's specific health problems.

4. _____ All health practitioners contribute to the problem list when a problem-oriented record format is used by a health agency.

5. _____ The initial plan of the patient's overall care needs does not have to include the patient's input.

6. _____ The PIE method of charting is the same as SOAP charting.

7. _____ Charting by exception is a method of check-list charting.

8. _____ The Patient's Bill of Rights states that the patient has the right to read his chart.

9. _____ One of the difficulties with computerized charting is patient confidentiality.
10. _____ The need to label time as AM or PM is eliminated by the use of military time.
11. _____ The nursing care plan is considered part of the patient's permanent record and is therefore a legal document.
12. _____ Information included on the Kardex should be written in ink.

SHORT ANSWER QUESTIONS

Directions: Read each of the following statements and supply the word(s) necessary in the space provided.

1. The analysis of the problem section of problem-oriented charting is called the _____

2. The section that states the effectiveness of the intervention in problem-oriented charting is called the
   _____

3. The information reported by the patient in problem-oriented charting is labeled _____

4. The section of the problem-oriented chart that shows the changes that will be made in the original plan is called _____

5. The section of the problem-oriented chart that gives the observations made by health personnel is called _____

CRITICAL THINKING EXERCISES

1. What type of records are used in the health agency where you work or study?
   a. _____ Traditional records
   b. _____ Problem-oriented records
   Briefly describe the differences between traditional records and problem-oriented records.

2. Refer to the sample nursing care plan (Figure 9-7) in Timby text. Identify the data you would expect to find in SOAP charting based on this plan of care.

C H A P T E R   1 0

Admission, Discharge, Transfer, and Referrals

SUMMARY

At some point in time most of us experience changes in health. Some become ill suddenly; some become injured; others may have felt ill for a while. All may need some form of care and treatment for their illness. To receive this treatment, we may be required to enter a health care agency such as a hospital or nursing home. The nurse faces a challenge to carry out agency policies for admission, transfer, referral, or discharge while helping the individual maintain his dignity and sense of control.

The information in this chapter is intended to assist the nursing student to understand and respond to the typical reactions that occur when a person is admitted to a hospital. Skill procedures that describe the general routines for admission and discharge of patients are also included. Methods for adapting these procedures to specific patient situations are discussed.

MATCHING QUESTIONS

Directions: For items 1 through 7, match the services listed in Part B with the organizations in Part A.

Part A

1. _____ Hospice
2. _____ Home-health aid
3. _____ Respite care
4. _____ Adult protective services
5. _____ Commission on aging
6. _____ Homemaker services
7. _____ Visiting nurses' association

Part B

a. Assists elderly with transportation to medical appointments, outpatient therapy, and community meal sites
b. Supports the family and terminally ill individuals who choose to stay at home
c. Offers intermittent nursing care to homebound persons
d. Provides one hot meal, sometimes two, per day either delivered at home or at a community meal site
e. Sends adults to the home to assist in shopping, meal preparation, and light housekeeping
f. Assists with bathing, hygiene, and medication supervision
g. Makes social, legal, and accounting services available to incompetent adults who may be victimized by others
h. Provides short-term, temporary relief to full-time caregivers of homebound persons
i. Investigates and resolves complaints made by, or on behalf of, nursing home residents

MULTIPLE CHOICE QUESTIONS

Directions: For items 1 through 10 circle the letter that corresponds to the best answer for each question.

1. An extended care facility licensed to provide skilled care is allowed to:
   a. Have nursing assistants give most of the care
   b. Give wound care, tube feedings, and intravenous fluids
   c. Arrange for room and board and carry out daily supervision
   d. Arrange social and recreational activities

2. Mr. J. was admitted through the emergency room after suffering a heart attack while on an out-of-town business trip. He asks the nurse to take his wallet for safekeeping. The best method of carrying out Mr. J.'s request is:
    a. Count the money with him and then tell him that you are placing his wallet in a locked drawer at the nurse's station.
    b. Count the money in front of him, have him sign a statement, and then place the statement on his chart.
    c. Tell him you will have someone from the business office come to collect his valuables and place them in the safe.
    d. Tell him that the hospital cannot be responsible for that much money and he will have to hide it.

3. The primary concern to the nurse when referring a patient is:
    a. Arranging transportation for the patient
    b. Notifying the agency that will receive the patient
    c. Communicating the information to the patient
    d. Getting everything organized so there is continuity of care

4. Discharge planning for the hospitalized patient begins:
    a. When the patient's physician gives the discharge order
    b. When the patient is admitted to the health care agency
    c. When the patient begins to ask about his discharge plans
    d. When all of the specific needs of the patient have been identified

5. When a rational adult wishes to leave the hospital against medical advice, which of the following is true:
    a. He may not leave until the physician examines him
    b. He may leave only after he has signed a special form
    c. He may leave because he cannot be forcefully detained
    d. He may leave after his attorney obtains permission

6. The nurse's responsibility when a patient wishes to leave the hospital against medical advice is:
    a. The nurse should explain to the patient that he may leave after being seen by her physician
    b. The nurse responsible for the patient's care should be sure the physician is notified and aware of the patient's wishes
    c. The nurse should note the request on the patient's record and have the patient sign a special form.
    d. The hospital administrator or the supervising nurse should notify the physician that his patient has left the agency.

7. Ordinarily the procedure after the patient has been discharged is:
    a. The nurse should clean and sterilize all of the equipment in the room
    b. The nurse should notify the housekeeping department that the patient has been discharged
    c. The nurse should notify the sterile supply personnel so that they may clean the used equipment
    d. The nurse should notify the administration office so the room will be cleaned properly

8. The term continuity of care means:
    a. Care provided in the home by home health aides after discharge
    b. Care that is not interrupted by a change in caregivers
    c. Care provided in a skilled, intermediate, or basic care facility
    d. Care that does not require the services offered in a nursing home

9. The process that occurs when a patient leaves a health care agency is called:
    a. Discharge
    b. Transfer
    c. Referral
    d. Admission

10. Which of the following statements best describes an intermediate care facility?
    a. An institution that provides health care for persons unable to care for themselves but who do not require hospitalization
    b. An institution that provides health services to persons who, because of mental or physical conditions, require care
    c. An institution that provides custodial care in a group setting to persons who can perform their own activities of daily living
    d. An institution that provides 24-hour nursing care under the direction of a registered nurse

TRUE OR FALSE QUESTIONS

Directions: For items 1 through 10, decide if the statement is true or false and mark T or F in the space provided.

1. _____ It is the nurse's responsibility to maintain the individual's sense of control and dignity during admission, transfer, referral, and discharge.

2. _____ Home health care services can be used to prevent hospital admission.

3. _____ Preparing an identification bracelet for the patient is one of the least important components of the admission process.

4. _____ The nurse should wait until the patient arrives on the unit before checking to make sure the room is prepared.

5. _____ One of the most important steps of the admission procedure is to make the patient feel welcome.

6. _____ Most hospital admission departments supply the patient with a policy booklet so that it is not necessary for the nurse to do the orientation.

7. _____ Losing personal items belonging to a patient can have serious implications unless there has been a signed and witnessed inventory that was taken at the time of admission.

8. _____ The transfer of a patient from one hospital unit to another should be handled in the same manner as discharging him from the one unit and admitting him to another.

9. _____ A step-down unit is often used for those patients who need long-term care or are terminally ill.

10. _____ A patient may be referred by a nurse in a hospital to outside organizations.

SHORT ANSWER QUESTION

List six of the guidelines for "Transferring a Patient" suggested in this chapter.

a. _____

b. _____

c. _____

d. _____

e. _____

f. _____

CRITICAL THINKING EXERCISES

1. Describe adjustments made in relation to admitting and discharging patients:
   a. When the patient is an infant or child

   b. When the patient is elderly

2. Plan a teaching program for the patient(s) for whom you are caring and complete the following form.

Topic for Teaching	Points to Cover in the Teaching Program
The hospital environment	
Preparation for discharge	

PERFORMANCE CHECKLIST

A. This section allows you to examine your techniques for assisting the patient with admission to a health care agency.

1. Place a check mark in the "S" ("satisfactory") column if you used the recommended technique.
2. Place a check mark in the "N.I." ("needs improvement") column if you used some but not all of each recommended technique.
3. Place a check mark in the "U" ("unsatisfactory") column if you forgot to include that particular recommended technique.
4. The section for comment allows space to make notes about when further practice is indicated, what errors you made, suggestions that will improve your skills, and so on.

Recommended Technique	S	N.I.	U	Comments
Check the patient's identification and greet him courteously				
Provide privacy to allow for undressing				
Assist the patient with undressing as indicated				
Care for clothing and valuables according to agency policy				
Explain hospital routines and policies				
Place signal device for the convenience of the patient				
Begin indicated care and document procedure				

B. Examine your techniques when discharging a patient from a health agency and complete the following form.

Recommended Technique	S	N.I.	U	Comments
Note that the patient has an order to be discharged				
See to it that the patient or a family member has discharge instructions				
See to it that the patient has necessary supplies and equipment for care				
Check to see that proper financial arrangements have been made				
Help the patient dress and see to it that transportation is available				
Document appropriately				

(continued)

C. Examine your techniques after referring a patient to another health agency and complete the following form.

Recommended Technique	S	N.I.	U	Comments
Note that the patient has an order for referral				
Note that the patient's identifying information is complete				
State the patient's diagnosis				
Describe the patient's disabilities, if any				
List the patient's diet and medications and include a medication schedule				
List the patient's allergies				
Include recent laboratory reports, if any				
Suggest appropriate exercise and activities				
State how the patient is to get to the agency and when he is to arrive				
Notify the agency of the patient's expected time of arrival				
Give a copy of this information to the patient or family member				
Direct the patient or family member to the appropriate person for help with financial arrangements				
Assist the patient to his transportation if appropriate				
Document appropriately				

PERFORMANCE CHECKLIST

This section allows you to examine your techniques for obtaining the patient's vital signs.

1. Place a check mark in the "S" ("satisfactory") column if you used the recommended technique.
2. Place a check mark in the "N.I." ("needs improvement") column if you used some but not all of each recommended technique.
3. Place a check mark in the "U" ("unsatisfactory") column if you forgot to include that particular recommended technique.
4. The section for comment allows space to make notes about when further practice is indicated, what errors you made, suggestions that will improve your skills, and so on.

Recommended Technique	S	N.I.	U	Comments
Obtaining an Oral Temperature				
Rinse thermometer that is stored in a chemical solution				
Wipe the thermometer while moving tissue from the bulb toward your fingers				
Shake thermometer down and read it at eye level to check that it is at its lowest marking				
Place the thermometer at the base and under the patient's tongue				
Leave the thermometer in place preferably 7 to 10 minutes but no less than 3 minutes				
Remove the thermometer and wipe it clean while moving tissue from your fingers toward the bulb				
Hold thermometer at eye level, read it, and then shake it down				
Follow agency policy to clean and store the thermometer				
Obtaining a Rectal Temperature				
Rinse a thermometer that is stored in a chemical solution				
Wipe thermometer while moving tissue from the bulb toward the fingers				
Shake the thermometer down and read it at eye level to check that it is at its lowest marking				

(continued)

Recommended Technique	S	N.I.	U	Comments
Lubricate the bulb and about 2.5 cm (1 inch) of the thermometer stem and fold back bed linens to expose anus				
Separate buttocks, insert the thermometer about 3.75 to 5 cm (1.5 to 2 inches), and allow buttocks to fall into place				
Hold the thermometer in place for 2 to 3 minutes				
Remove the thermometer and wipe it clean while moving tissue from your fingers toward the bulb				
Hold the thermometer at eye level, read it, and then shake it down				
Follow agency policy to clean and store the thermometer				
Obtaining an Axillary Temperature				
Rinse a thermometer that is stored in a chemical solution				
Wipe the thermometer while moving the tissue from the bulb toward your fingers				
Shake the thermometer down and read it at eye level to check that it is at its lowest marking				
Place the thermometer well into the axillary region with the bulb directed toward the patient's head				
Bring the patient's arm down close to the body and place his forearm over his chest toward the opposite shoulder				
Leave the thermometer in place for 10 minutes, preferably 15 minutes				
Remove the thermometer and wipe it clean while moving tissue from your fingers toward the bulb				
Hold the thermometer at eye level, read it, and then shake it down				
Follow agency policy to clean and store the thermometer				
Obtaining the Radial Pulse Rate				
If the patient is lying down, place the patient's arm alongside his body, wrist extended, palm of hand downward				

Recommended Technique	S	N.I.	U	Comments
If patient is sitting, place forearm at about a 90° angle to his body, forearm extended, palm of hand downward				
Place three fingertips along the radial artery while the thumb rests on the back of the patient's wrist				
Press gently to close the artery and then slowly release pressure until the pulse can be felt				
While using a watch with a sweep secondhand, count the pulse for ½ minute and multiply by 2				
If pulse is abnormal, count the pulse for at least 1 full minute, longer if necessary for accuracy				
Obtaining the Respiratory Rate				
While the fingertips are in place after counting the pulse rate, observe the patient's respirations				
Note each rise and fall of the patient's chest wall as she breathes				
While using a watch with a sweep secondhand, count the respiratory rate for ½ minute and multiply by 2				
If respirations are abnormal, count the respirations for at lease 1 minute, longer if necessary for accuracy				
Obtaining the Blood Pressure with a Mercury Manometer at the Brachial Artery				
Delay taking the blood pressure, except in an emergency, if the patient is upset, is in pain, or has just exercised				
Have the patient comfortable, with the forearm supported at the level of the heart, palm upward, and upper arm extended				
Have the patient seated so that the meniscus of mercury can be read at eye level and no more than 3 feet away from the manometer				
Place a cuff of appropriate size so that the inflatable bag is centered over the brachial artery				
Have the lower edge of the cuff about 2.5 to 5 cm (1 to 2 inches) above the inner aspect of the elbow				
Have the rubber tubing leaving the cuff at the edge nearer to the patient's elbow				

(continued)

Recommended Technique	S	N.I.	U	Comments
Wrap cuff smoothly and snugly and secure it in place				
Feel for the brachial artery after placing the stethoscope earpieces in your ears				
Place stethoscope disk over the artery where the pulse was felt, away from clothes and the cuff				
Pump air into the cuff to an amount about 30 mmHg above the point where the radial pulse disappears				
Release air gradually with the valve on the bulb, 2 to 3 mmHg per heartbeat				
Note the reading on the manometer when the first two consecutive heartbeats are heard; note this as systolic pressure				
Continue releasing air; note when a distinct, soft, muffling sound is heard; note this as diastolic pressure				
Observe when all sounds disappear and note this as the third reading; this may occur at the same time as diastole				
Allow remaining air to escape from the cuff quickly and remove the cuff from the patient's arm				
Clean and store equipment according to agency policy				
Obtaining the Radial-Apical Pulse				
While working with a second nurse, expose the patient's left chest wall				
First nurse: Place stethoscope disk over the apical area of the heart and listen for the pulse beat				
Second nurse: Place fingertips over the radial artery and feel for the pulse beat				
Second nurse: Hold watch with a sweep secondhand so that both nurses can read it				
Select a starting time and both nurses count pulse beats for 1 minute, longer if necessary for accuracy				

PERFORMANCE CHECKLIST

This section allows you to examine your techniques for performing a physical assessment.

1. Place a check mark in the "S" ("satisfactory") column if you used the recommended technique.
2. Place a check mark in the "N.I." ("needs improvement") column if you used some but not all of each recommended technique.
3. Place a check mark in the "U" ("unsatisfactory") column if you forgot to include that particular recommended technique.
4. The section for comment allows space to make notes about when further practice is indicated, what errors you made, suggestions that will improve your skills, and so on.

Recommended Technique	S	N.I.	U	Comments
Identify the patient				
Explain what is planned				
Assemble the equipment needed				
Provide privacy during the examination				
Wash your hands before beginning the examination				
Assist the patient in putting on an examining gown				
Provide a cover for other exposed areas				
Explain that all information will be kept confidential				
Raise the bed or examination table to a comfortable working height				
Protect the patient from injury				
Follow the health agency's policy for the examination				
Explain each technique before it is performed				
Proceed through the examination in an organized manner				
Review your data				
Assist the patient as needed upon completion of the examination				

(continued)

Recommended Technique	S	N.I.	U	Comments
Make sure that all equipment is cleaned or replaced				
Record the assessment information				
Communicate any significant information to the appropriate nursing or medical personnel				

CHAPTER 13

Special Examinations and Tests

SUMMARY

This chapter gives a general overview of nursing responsibilities associated with assisting with examinations and special tests. These are performed to determine how the body is functioning and are carried out by various health care personnel. Often, the nurse is required to prepare the patient both physically and emotionally for the test or examination, assist with the procedure itself, and care for the patient and equipment afterward. In addition, several possible nursing diagnoses are suggested for patients undergoing tests and examinations. An example of the nursing process as it relates to one of these diagnoses is included in the nursing care plan.

MATCHING QUESTIONS

Directions: For items 1 through 5, match the descriptions of the common positions for examinations and tests in Part B with the names of the positions in Part A.

Part A
1. _____ Modified standing
2. _____ Dorsal recumbent
3. _____ Lithotomy
4. _____ Sim's
5. _____ Genupectoral

Part B
a. The patient is lying on his back with the feet in stirrups and the buttocks at the edge of the table end
b. The patient assumes the normal standing position with arms relaxed at the sides
c. The patient rests on her knees and chest. The head is turned to one side and the arms are above the head

d. The patient is lying on his back with the legs separated and the knees bent so the feet are flat against the table or bed
e. The patient is lying on her side
f. The buttocks are firmly on the edge of the bed. Most of the thighs are supported and the feet are on the floor or on a foot rest
g. The patient is standing in front of and facing the examination table, leaning forward from the waist

Directions: For items 6 through 13, match the descriptions of the tests or examinations in Part B with the names of the tests in Part A.

Part A
6. _____ Roentgenography
7. _____ Magnetic resonance
8. _____ Computed tomography
9. _____ Electromyography
10. _____ Ultrasonography
11. _____ Positron emission tomography
12. _____ Endoscopy
13. _____ Biopsy

Part B
a. Uses sound waves to produce images on a screen
b. Uses x-rays to produce images
c. Uses x-rays plus contrast medium to identify variations in tissue density
d. Sniping a piece of tissue for examination
e. Uses electrical impulses from skeletal muscles to produce wave patterns
f. Scans magnetic forces with radio-frequency signals
g. Combines radionuclide scanning and layered tomography
h. Uses an instrument for visual examination of an internal structure

MULTIPLE CHOICE QUESTIONS

Directions: For items 1 through 12, circle the letter that corresponds to the best answer for each question.

1. The suffix–ogram refers to which of the following:
    a. An examination in which body structures are visualized by the eye
    b. The procedure in which an image of a particular body part is produced
    c. The instrument used to visualize a particular part of the body
    d. The actual image or results of the test that may be held in the hand

2. The suffix–centesis refers to which of the following:
    a. When a procedure involves puncturing a body cavity
    b. When a procedure involves producing an image of a body part
    c. When a procedure involves visualizing an area within the body
    d. When a procedure involves the production of a paper strip of waves

3. Paracentesis is best described as:
    a. The removal of fluid from the lungs, bronchi, and trachea via the introduction of a bronchoscope
    b. The removal of fluid or air from the pleural cavity by entering the thorax through the chest wall
    c. The removal of secretions from the stomach after the insertion of a nasogastric tube
    d. The removal of body fluid by puncturing the skin and subsequently the abdominal cavity

4. The reason for a Queckenstedt's test is:
    a. To determine if there is an obstruction in the spinal canal
    b. To determine if there is an infection in the spinal canal
    c. To determine the amount of fluid in the spinal canal
    d. To determine the amount of pressure in the spinal canal

5. Of the following which is used to determine the activity of the brain:
    a. Electrocardiography
    b. Electromyography
    c. Electroencephalography
    d. Echocardiography

6. The dorsal recumbent position is most often used to examine:
    a. The heart and lungs
    b. The rectum and vagina
    c. The rectum and colon
    d. The bladder and uterus

7. The lithotomy position is most often used to examine:
    a. The heart and lungs
    b. The rectum and vagina
    c. The rectum and colon
    d. The bladder and uterus

8. Which of the following are the three essential elements of informed consent:
    a. Capacity, consent, comprehension
    b. Ability, coercion, risks
    c. Rationality, explanation, alternatives
    d. Capacity, comprehension, voluntariness

9. A cystoscopy refers to an examination that involves:
    a. Inspection of the bronchi
    b. Inspection of the abdominal cavity
    c. Inspection of the colon
    d. Inspection of the urinary bladder

10. The modified standing position is most commonly used to:
    a. Insert a suppository
    b. Complete a cystoscopic examination
    c. Examine the prostate gland
    d. Collect a Pap smear

11. On the cellular portion of the Pap smear, a Class III result would indicate:
    a. The result is negative with no abnormal cells
    b. The result is suggestive of cancer cells; it is not definite
    c. The result is strongly suggestive of cancer cells
    d. The result is definitely cancerous cells

12. On the identifiable microorganisms portion of the Pap smear, a #1 result would indicate:
    a. Normal microorganisms
    b. Scanty microorganisms
    c. Trichomonas vaginalis
    d. Monilia

TRUE OR FALSE QUESTIONS

Directions: For items 1 through 15, decide if the statement is true or false and mark T or F in the space provided.

1. _____ The physician is responsible for explaining an invasive procedure.

2. _____ It is important that the nurse memorize all the special requirements for the various tests and examinations that are performed.

3. _____ The nurse is usually responsible for obtaining the necessary equipment when special diagnostic examinations and tests are performed on the nursing unit.

4. _____ Draping is done prior to an examination to prevent the patient from becoming chilled.

5. _____ All patients should be asked about allergies prior to tests and examinations that use contrast media.

6. _____ When iodine is altered in such a way that it gives off radiation, it is referred to as a gamma ray.

7. _____ Ultrasonography can be used to examine moving structures, such as the heart or a fetus.

8. _____ A spinal tap is a procedure in which a needle is inserted between lumbar vertebrae in the spine but below the spinal cord itself in order to obtain spinal fluid.

9. _____ Examinations using x-rays or radionuclides should not be performed on pregnant or breast-feeding women.

10. _____ Alcohol is the best cleaning agent for cleansing the skin when preparing the area for a blood glucose test.

11. _____ To produce an accurate blood glucose test, the test strip pad must be completely covered and saturated with blood.

12. _____ A preliminary diagnosis may be obtained from a throat culture in 10 minutes.

13. _____ Glucose and insulin are hormones that regulate carbohydrate metabolism in the body.

14. _____ Blood sugar is usually measured one-half hour before eating a meal and before bedtime to determine the lowest level of glucose in the blood.

15. _____ A signoidoscopy involves inspecting the rectum and a section of the lower intestine with an endoscope.

SHORT ANSWER QUESTIONS

Directions: Read each of the following statements and supply the word(s) necessary in the space provided.

1. List six items of information that should be included in a patient's record regarding an examination or special test that has been performed.
   a. _____
   b. _____
   c. _____
   d. _____
   e. _____
   f. _____

2. Identify three factors to be considered when examinations and tests are performed on older adults.
   a. _____
   b. _____
   c. _____

3. Name five patient responsibilities that should be included in a teaching plan for patients receiving tests or examinations on an out-patient basis.
   a. _____
   b. _____
   c. _____
   d. _____
   e. _____

CRITICAL THINKING EXERCISE

Describe nursing responsibilities for a pregnant woman who is having an amniocentesis (withdrawal of a sample of amniotic fluid for testing). How would the sample be cared for?

PERFORMANCE CHECKLIST

This section allows you to examine your techniques for assisting with examinations and special tests.

1. Place a check mark in the "S" ("satisfactory") column if you used the recommended technique.
2. Place a check mark in the "N.I." ("needs improvement") column if you used some but not all of each recommended technique.
3. Place a check mark in the "U" ("unsatisfactory") column if you forgot to include that particular recommended technique.
4. The section for comment allows space to make notes about when further practice is indicated, what errors you made, suggestions that will improve your skills, and so on.

Recommended Technique	S	N.I.	U	Comments
Understand the nature of the procedure, why it is being done, what part of the body is to be entered, and the specimen to be collected				
Understand the patient, the diagnosis, and the plan of care				
Prepare the patient psychologically for the procedure				
Obtain a permit if one is required				
Have the patient void prior to the procedure				
Gown the patient properly				
The patient's skin at the site of entry should be clean and shaved if necessary				
Validate that special preparations have been carried out for the procedure				
Have the necessary equipment and supplies ready. Equipment is in working order				
Prepare the working area and position and drape the patient appropriately				
Clean the skin at the site of entry and handle equipment, as required, to assist the examiner				
Care for the patient appropriately after the procedure is completed				
Assist an examiner appropriately when he or she carries out the following:				

(continued)

Recommended Technique	S	N.I.	U	Comments
A lumbar puncture				
A thoracentesis				
An abdominal paracentesis				

CHAPTER 14

Nutrition

SUMMARY

Nutrition is a basic human need. If a person is deprived of food for a prolonged period of time, health will be affected and life may be endangered. Most eating habits are learned early in life and usually vary from culture to culture. Research data supports the idea that nutritional status has a great influence on health and well being. Modifying and regulating food intake are standard techniques used in the treatment of illness.

Nurses should possess certain skills that enable them to assist the patient to obtain adequate nutrition within the limits of his illness. Several skills and guidelines are included for this purpose.

MATCHING QUESTIONS

Directions: For items 1 through 5, match the chief functions in Part B with the common minerals needed by the body in Part A.

Part A
1. _____ Sodium
2. _____ Potassium
3. _____ Calcium
4. _____ Iodine
5. _____ Iron

Part B
a. Buffering action and the formation of bones and teeth
b. Neuromuscular activity, blood coagulation, cell wall permeability, and formation of teeth and bones
c. Activation of enzymes, neuromuscular activity, and formation of teeth and bones
d. Maintenance of water and electrolyte balance
e. Component of hemoglobin and assistance in cellular oxidation
f. Enzyme reactions, neuromuscular activity, and maintenance of fluid and electrolyte balance

g. Regulation of body metabolism and promotion of normal growth

Directions: For items 6 through 8, match the vitamins in Part B with the deficiency diseases in Part A.

6. _____ Scurvy
7. _____ Rickets
8. _____ Beriberi

Part B
a. Vitamin A
b. Vitamin B
c. Vitamin C
d. Vitamin D
e. Vitamin E

Directions: For items 9 through 13, match the characteristics in Part B with the types of diets in Part A.

Part A
9. _____ Regular/standard
10. _____ Soft
11. _____ Mechanical soft
12. _____ Full liquid
13. _____ Clear liquid

Part B
a. A light diet used for patients with chewing difficulties; provides cooked fruits and vegetables and ground meats
b. A wide variety, such as high-caloric, low-caloric, diabetic, restricted sodium, low-fat, high-protein, and low-roughage diets
c. Allows unrestricted food selections
d. Contains fruit and vegetable juices, creamed or blended soups, milk, ices, ice cream, gelatin, junket, custard and cooked cereal
e. Primarily a regular diet with the omission of fried foods, rich pastries, fat-rich foods, and gas-forming and raw foods

63

f. Consists of water, clear broth, clear fruit juice, plain gelatin, tea and coffee, may or may not include carbonated beverages

g. Contains foods soft in texture, usually low in residue and easily digestible, few or no spices, few fruits, vegetables, or meats

MULTIPLE CHOICE QUESTIONS

Directions: For items 1 through 16, circle the letter that corresponds to the best answer for each question.

1. Which of the following best describes nutrition:
    a. The body's need for calories, water, proteins, carbohydrates, fats, vitamins, and minerals
    b. The process whereby the body uses food and fluids to reach and maintain health
    c. The comparison of a certain volume or weight of the energy source with its ability to produce heat
    d. Food is a source of body energy for human beings, and it provides the means by which human beings function

2. A calorie is defined as the amount of heat necessary to raise the temperature of:
    a. 1 pound of water by 1° F
    b. 1 pound of water by 1° C
    c. 1 gram of water by 1° F
    d. 1 gram of water by 1° C

3. The average adult requirement of calories per day is:
    a. 1000–2000
    b. 1500–2500
    c. 2000–3000
    d. 3000–4000

4. Of the following substances, which supplies the body with amino acids:
    a. Proteins
    b. Fats
    c. Carbohydrates
    d. Minerals

5. The caloric yield of fats is:
    a. 4 calories per gram
    b. 5 calories per gram
    c. 7 calories per gram
    d. 9 calories per gram

6. The recommended percentage of dietary fat per day is:
    a. 10%
    b. 20%
    c. 30%
    d. 15%

7. Which of the following provide the body with necessary electrolytes:
    a. Vitamins
    b. Proteins
    c. Minerals
    d. Fats

8. Individuals who eat vegetarian diets maybe lacking:
    a. Amino acids
    b. Vitamins
    c. Electrolytes
    d. Iron

9. Regurgitation commonly occurs in which of the following age groups:
    a. The elderly
    b. The toddler
    c. The infant
    d. The adolescent

10. The person with anorexia may feel most like eating at:
    a. Breakfast time
    b. Lunchtime
    c. Dinner time
    d. Bedtime

11. Which of the following lipoproteins carry cholesterol to cells and tissue:
    a. Very low-density lipoproteins
    b. Low-density lipoproteins
    c. High-density lipoproteins
    d. Very high-density lipoproteins

12. Among lipoproteins, a major source of low-density lipoproteins is:
    a. Triglycerides
    b. Cholesterol
    c. Very low-density lipoproteins
    d. Very high-density lipoproteins

13. Which of the following represents the normal range of measurement for the triceps skin fold in adult males?
    a. 29.3–17.6 cm
    b. 25.3–15.2 cm
    c. 16.5–9.90 mm
    d. 12.5–7.5 mm

14. Minerals are best described as:
    a. Non-caloric substances that are essential to all cells
    b. Chemical substances that are necessary in minute amounts
    c. Substances that contain as much hydrogen as their molecules can hold
    d. Chemical compounds composed of nitrogen, carbon, hydrogen, and oxygen

15. The term dysphagia refers to:
    a. Difficulty swallowing
    b. Impairment of intellectual function
    c. Desire to vomit
    d. Discharge of gas through the mouth

16. Good sources of carbohydrates in food are:
    a. Grains, meat, fish, eggs, tomatoes
    b. Eggs, milk, avocados, nuts, chocolate
    c. Cereals, grains, wheat germ, fruits, vegetables
    d. Seafood, potatoes, soup, peanut butter, corn

TRUE OR FALSE QUESTIONS

Directions: For items 1 through 10, decide if the statement is true or false and mark T or F in the space provided.

1. _____ An individual's eating habits are determined primarily by hereditary factors.
2. _____ Anorexia is defined, as a condition in which there is a general wasting away of body tissue.
3. _____ The synonym for eructation is belching.
4. _____ Flatus refers to intestinal gas released from the rectum.
5. _____ Protein complementation is the combining of animal and plant sources in the same meal.
6. _____ The bulk that helps with elimination comes from the undigestible fiber found in the stems, skins, and leaves of many fruits and vegetables.
7. _____ Many deficiency diseases have been associated with diets in which specific foods, rich in a source of fats, have been lacking.
8. _____ Water-soluble vitamins are stored in the body as reserve for future needs.
9. _____ Consuming megadoses of vitamins can be dangerous.
10. _____ Strict vegetarians should take vitamin B supplements.

SHORT ANSWER QUESTIONS

Directions: Read each of the following statements and supply the word(s) necessary in the space provided.

1. List the six basic food groups and state the number of servings per day for each.

Food Group	Servings per Day
a. _____	_____
b. _____	_____
c. _____	_____
d. _____	_____
e. _____	_____
f. _____	_____

2. Describe three facts that can be obtained from a current nutritional label.
   a. _____
   b. _____
   c. _____

CRITICAL THINKING EXERCISES

1. Prepare a three-day menu plan for an economically disadvantaged couple. The wife is 72 and has arthritis. The husband is 74 and has Alzheimer's disease. They are able to consume a regular diet. However, the husband has loose fitting dentures and often can not remember where he put them. They have no close family. Consider community resources in your area for transportation, shopping, and meal preparation.

2. Prepare a one-day menu plan for a child vegetarian. The meals should meet the recommended daily allowance of essential nutrients for this child.

3. Identify daily medications taken by a client you have cared for. Describe dietary considerations for each of these medications. Discuss how the client would plan to satisfy these conditions.

PERFORMANCE CHECKLIST

A. This section allows you to examine your techniques for assisting the patient to eat and for assisting to serve meals to hospitalized patients.

1. Place a check mark in the "S" ("satisfactory") column if you used the recommended technique.
2. Place a check mark in the "N.I." ("needs improvement") column if you used some but not all of each recommended technique

3. Place a check mark in the "U" ("unsatisfactory") column if you forgot to include that particular recommended technique.
4. The section for comment allows space to make notes about when further practice is indicated, what errors you made, suggestions that will improve your skills, and so on.

Recommended Technique	S	N.I.	U	Comments
Plan ahead so that a period of rest and measures to relieve pain are provided before mealtime				
Avoid giving treatments immediately before or after meals				
Use available measures to help control noise and odors before mealtimes				
See to it that the room is tidy before the meal is served				
Offer the patient a bedpan or urinal before serving a meal				
Offer the patient equipment and supplies to wash her hands; give oral hygiene as indicated				
Provide privacy for seriously ill patients who cannot eat				
Assist the patient to a comfortable and safe position for eating				
Check to see that the correct tray and foods are served to the patient				
See to it that the tray is complete, tidy, and promptly served				
Protect the patient and bed linens with a napkin				
Sit at the patient's bedside while helping her to eat				

(continued)

Recommended Technique	S	N.I.	U	Comments
Encourage the patient to help herself with eating, as indicated				
Serve manageable bits of food in the order of the patient's preference; offer fluids intermittently				
Allow the patient adequate time to chew and swallow				
Note foods the patient is not eating, see to it that the patient has sufficient food, and report accordingly				
Offer support to patients who may not enjoy a special diet				
Keep conversation friendly during mealtimes				
When a patient has limited eyesight, devise a system to indicate when she is ready for more food				
Remove trays promptly after meals and offer oral hygiene and an opportunity for the patient to wash her hands				
Leave the patient clean and comfortable				

B. Examine your techniques while caring for a patient when anorexia, nausea, and vomiting are present and complete the following form.

Recommended Technique	S	N.I.	U	Comments
Control odors, noises, and annoying sights as much as possible				
Avoid making negative comments about food				
Limit the patient's activities appropriately				
Use deep-breathing exercises to help the patient control her nausea and vomiting				
Limit food and fluid intake appropriately when nausea and vomiting are present				
Offer the patient bland foods and avoid spicy and high-fat foods				
Use carbonated beverages and ice chips appropriately to relieve nausea and vomiting				
Use appropriate measures to prevent vomitus from being aspirated, including using suction if necessary				

Recommended Technique	S	N.I.	U	Comments
After the patient vomits, help with oral hygiene				
After the patient vomits, wash her hands and face, change linens, and give the patient a backrub				
See to it that the patient is in a comfortable position and in a quiet environment after nausea and vomiting				

PERFORMANCE CHECKLIST

A. This section allows you to examine your techniques for controlling oral fluid intake.
1. Place a check mark in the "S" ("satisfactory") column if you used the recommended technique.
2. Place a check mark in the "N.I." ("needs improvement") column if you used some but not all of each recommended technique.
3. Place a check mark in the "U" ("unsatisfactory") column if you forgot to include that particular recommended technique.

4. The section for comment allows space to make notes about when further practice is indicated, what errors you made, suggestions that will improve your skills, and so on.

Examine your techniques when a patient is to have fluids encouraged and when one is to have fluids restricted and complete the following form.

Recommended Technique	S	N.I.	U	Comments
Fluid Intake Increase				
Keep fluid handy at the bedside at all times				
Offer a variety of fluids				
Set goals with the patient for amount of fluid to take				
Offer foods, as permitted, having high water content				
Serve fluids at their proper temperature				
Offer proportionately more fluids early in the day				
Fluid Intake Decrease				
Keep fluid out of sight as much as possible				
Use small containers for serving fluids				
Avoid serving foods that tend to increase thirst				
Set goals with the patient for spacing allowable fluids				
Use various techniques to maintain good oral hygiene				
Offer ice chips, as allowed				

(continued)

B. This section allows you to examine your techniques for initiating an intravenous infusion.

Recommended Technique	S	N.I.	U	Comments
Assemble appropriate equipment and supplies, including the solution				
Select an appropriate and accessible vein for injecting				
Use appropriate techniques when a vein cannot be felt: Have the patient lower his arm and make a fist—open and close fist				
Gently tap over the vein				
Place warm, moist compresses on the vein				
Stroke the skin toward the fingers				
Place the arm on a supportive surface				
Tie the tourniquet 2 to 4 inches above the site of entry with its ends away from the site and clean the site correctly				
Stabilize the vein and soft tissue with the thumb				
Hold the needle, bevel side up, at a 45° angle above or to the side of the vein				
Pierce the vein and insert the needle about $\frac{1}{8}$ to $\frac{1}{4}$ inch				
When blood comes back through the needle, release the tourniquet and start the flow of solution				
Support and secure the catheter in place and adjust the flow of solution to the prescribed rate				
Monitor the intravenous infusion regularly and regulate the rate of flow as necessary				
Observe the patient for complications and report unusual signs/symptoms promptly				
Discontinue the infusion properly when the prescribed amount of solution has entered the vein				

C. This section allows you to examine your techniques for assisting with a blood transfusion.

Recommended Technique	S	N.I.	U	Comments
Identify the patient				
Take the patient's vital signs within 30 minutes of obtaining blood				

Recommended Technique	S	N.I.	U	Comments
Check and double-check with another person to be sure the proper blood is to be given to the correct patient				
Check to see that the blood has not passed its expiration date				
Be ready and prepared to give the blood as soon as it arrives from the blood bank				
Rotate the blood to mix the red blood cells; do not warm the blood				
At the bedside, check the information on the blood bag with patient information with another nurse				
Start the blood flow, turn off the saline solution				
Give the blood slowly, remain with the patient for at least 15 minutes. Observe for signs of a reaction (rate 2 ml per minute)				
If no signs of a reaction appear, increase the speed of flow to the prescribed rate (7–9 ml per minute)				
Continue to observe the patient for a reaction and stop giving blood when any sign of a reaction appears				
Assessments are done at 15- to 30-minute intervals				
Discontinue the blood transfusion in the same manner as an intravenous infusion when the blood is absorbed				

D. This section allows you to examine your techniques for changing solution containers.

Recommended Technique	S	N.I.	U	Comments
Determine that the solution to replace the current infusion is available				
Switch the containers when the infusing container is almost empty and the drip chamber still contains fluid				
Close the regulator on the tubing				
Remove the empty container and tubing from the standard				

(continued)

Recommended Technique	S	N.I.	U	Comments
Pull the spike from the current container without touching the tip				
Remove the seal from the replacement solution				
Immediately insert the spike into the replacement container				
Hang the new solution				
Inspect for the presence of air in the tubing and remove it				
Readjust the rate to the ordered or scheduled rate				
Record the volume of infused solution				
Record the addition of the new solution				

E. This section allows you to examine your techniques for changing infusion tubing.

Recommended Technique	S	N.I.	U	Comments
Obtain sterile infusion tubing like that being currently used				
Tighten the regulator clamp on the replacement tubing				
Remove the solution container from the standard				
Remove the outdated spike and replace it with the fresh, sterile spike using sterile technique				
Replace the solution on the standard				
Compress the drip chamber to fill it approximately ½ full				
Remove the protective cap from the other end and clear the tubing of air by loosening the regulator				
Close the regulator and replace the protective cap				
Peel back or remove the dressing over the venipuncture site				
Disconnect the outdated tubing while holding the venipuncture device firmly				
Remove the protective cap and attach the fresh, sterile tubing to the venipuncture device				
Loosen the regulator clamp and readjust the rate of flow				

Recommended Technique	S	N.I.	U	Comments
Label the tubing with the current date and time				
Record the procedure on the correct form				

F. This section allows you to examine your techniques for inserting an intermittent venous access device.

Recommended Technique	S	N.I.	U	Comments
Confirm the medication order to discontinue the continuous intravenous drip and insert a medication lock				
Inspect the site to determine if it can be maintained or if a new site is needed				
Assemble necessary equipment				
Explain the process to the patient				
Prefill chamber of medication lock with saline or heparin				
Loosen tape and expose the connection between the hub of the catheter and tubing adapter				
Loosen protective cap from the end of the medication lock				
Wear clean gloves				
Tighten the roller clamp to close or stop the infusion pump				
Apply pressure over catheter tip. Remove tip of tubing from venipuncture device and insert medication lock				
Swab rubber port on medication lock with alcohol				
Gradually instill 1 ml of saline or heparin				
Retape and secure the dressing				
Flush the lock with 1 or 2 ml of either saline or heparin flush solution after each use or at least every 8 hours				
Document assessment data, flush solution, discontinuation of continuous intravenous solution, date, and time				

CHAPTER 16

Hygiene

SUMMARY

Emphasis in this chapter is placed on nursing measures to promote personal hygiene. Personal cleanliness is an essential part of one's health care practices. When the individual is unable to care for himself, the nurse must possess the skills necessary to provide this aspect of care. The nurse functions in this area as a role model and health care teacher. She must assist the patient to differentiate between what is fact and what is fiction while continuing to be supportive of the patient's individual method of maintaining personal hygiene.

MATCHING QUESTIONS

Directions: For items 1 through 6, match the definitions in Part B with the terms in Part A:

Part A
1. ___D___ Bridge
2. ___e___ Caries
3. ___b___ Gingivitis
4. ___c___ Plaque
5. ___g___ Sordes
6. ___a___ Tartar

Part B
a. Hardened plaque
b. Inflammation of the gums
c. Mucin and grit in saliva
d. Dental appliance
e. Cavities
f. Baby teeth
g. Dried crust on the upper lips

Directions: The following substances may be used for oral care for items 7 through 10. Match the uses in Part B with the substances in Part A.

Part A
7. ___c___ Antiseptic mouthwash
E 8. ___D___ Hydrogen peroxide and water
B 9. ___e___ Lemon and glycerin swabs
10. ___f___ Petroleum jelly

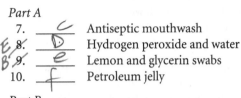

Part B
a. Reduces oral acidity
b. Increases salivation
c. Reduces bacterial growth
d. Removes accumulated secretions
e. Loosens dry, sticky particles
f. Lubricates lips

MULTIPLE CHOICE QUESTIONS

Directions: For items 1 through 14, circle the letter that corresponds to the best answer for each question.

1. The primary concern for nurses when assisting the patient with hygiene is:
   a. Personal care does not have to be carried out in an identical fashion for all patients
   b. Personal care should be carried out in a manner that promotes health for the individual
   c. The exact procedures as prescribed by the health agency must be followed when promoting hygiene
   d. The way in which personal care is promoted is not important, only that it must be done for the patient

2. The skin is the main component of which of the following systems:
   a. The immune system
   b. The muscular system
   c. The endocrine system
   d. The integumentary system

3. The oral hygiene practice recommended to break up bacteria lodged between the teeth is:
   a. Using dental floss between the teeth
   b. Directing a jet spray between the teeth
   c. Rinsing the mouth vigorously with a mouthwash
   d. Using an electric toothbrush regularly

4. Of the following procedures, which should be done first when toenails are thick and difficult to cut:
   a. File the rough edges first
   b. Soak the feet in warm water
   c. Massage a cream into the nails
   d. Apply an antiseptic to the nails

5. Which of the following is recommended when grooming hair that is tangled:
   a. Use a fine-toothed comb and start for the ends of the hair
   b. Use a wide-toothed comb and start near the scalp
   c. Use a fine-toothed comb and start near the scalp
   d. Use a wide-toothed comb and start from the ends of the hair

6. Which of the following types of glands found in the skin are responsible for regulating body temperature:
   a. Sudoriferous
   b. Ceruminous
   c. Sebaceous
   d. Ciliary

7. Immersion of the buttocks and perineum in a small basin of continuously circulating water is called a:
   a. Sponge bath
   b. Whirlpool bath
   c. Sitz bath
   d. Medicated bath

8. Of the following substances, which can be used for oral care to reduce oral acidity, dissolve plaque, and soothe oral lesions:
   a. Petroleum jelly
   b. Milk of magnesia
   c. Hydrogen peroxide
   d. Lemon and glycerin

9. An accumulation of cerumen within the ear may cause which of the following sound disturbances for patients with a hearing aid:
   a. Garbled sound
   b. Shrill feedback
   c. Increased noise
   d. Reduced sound

10. The temperature of the water for a tub bath should be:
    a. 105 to 110° F
    b. 110 to 115° F
    c. 90 to 105° F
    d. 100 to 105° F

11. The outermost layer of the skin is called:
    a. The dermis
    b. The keratin layer
    c. The epidermis
    d. The subcutaneous layer

12. In humans, the teeth begin to erupt at which of the following ages:
    a. 6 months of age
    b. 12 months of age
    c. 18 months of age
    d. 24 months of age

13. The term gingivitis refers to:
    a. Tooth decay
    b. Hardened plaque
    c. Inflammation of the jaws
    d. Inflammation of the gums

14. The term partial bath refers to:
    a. Washing the area around the patient's genitals and rectum only
    b. Washing in a manner to remove secretions and excretions from less soiled to more soiled areas
    c. Washing areas of the body that are subject to the greatest soiling or odor
    d. Washing all areas of the body at the sink in the patient's room

TRUE OR FALSE QUESTIONS

Directions: For items 1 through 12, decide if the statement is true or false and mark T or F in the space provided.

1. ___F___ It is safe to assume that patients with glasses are not also wearing contact lenses.

2. ___T___ Many health care agencies require that routine hygienic care be recorded in the nurse's notes.

3. __F__ A dental bridge is a prosthesis.
4. __F__ The nurse does not have to be tolerant of personal hygiene preferences when the patient is in the hospital.
5. __F__ Ceruminous glands secrete cerumen, a wax-like substance found in the external ear.
6. __F__ Hot water should be used when soaking a patient's dentures.
7. __T__ A physician's order should be obtained before cutting the toenails of patients with diabetes or vascular disease.
8. __T__ The use of preparations made with oil will help loosen tangled hair.
9. __T__ The subcutaneous layer separates the skin from skeletal muscle.
10. _____ Goblet cells located within the hair follicles release an oily substance called sebum.
11. _____ The texture, elasticity, and porosity of hair are inherited characteristics.
12. __T__ Fingernails and toenails acquire their tough texture from keratin.

SHORT ANSWER QUESTIONS

Directions: Read each of the following statements and supply the word(s) necessary in the space provided.

1. List four of the functions of the skin (as suggested in this chapter).
   a. _____
   b. _____
   c. _____
   d. _____

2. List four characteristics of healthy nails.
   a. _pink_
   b. _thin_
   c. _smooth_
   d. _skin @ nail be intact_
3. The usual number of permanent teeth in an adult mouth is _32_.
4. List four benefits of bathing
   a. _cleanse_
   b. _relaxation_
   c. _eliminates oder odor_
   d. _simulates infection_

CRITICAL THINKING EXERCISES

1. Complete this form below by writing a teaching plan for a patient in each of the following situations. List points to discuss in the teaching plan.

2. Review the nursing care plan included in this chapter. Recall an individual to whom you have recently been assigned. Using the components of the nursing process, develop a plan of care to meet the personal hygiene needs of this individual. Ask your clinical instructor to assist you.

Topic for Teaching	Points to Cover in a Teaching Plan
Measures to promote personal hygiene, as indicated, including when the patient is a diabetic.	
The prevention of tooth and gum diseases.	
Promoting personal hygiene when the patient is cared for at home.	

PERFORMANCE CHECKLIST

This section allows you to examine your techniques for assisting the patient with personal hygiene.

1. Place a check mark in the "S" ("satisfactory") column if you used the recommended technique.
2. Place a checkmark in the "N.I." ("needs improvement") column if you used some but not all of each recommended technique.
3. Place a check mark in the "U" ("unsatisfactory") column if you forgot to include that particular recommended technique.
4. The section for comment allows space to make notes about when further practice is indicated, what errors you made, suggestions that will improve your skills, and so on.

Recommended Technique	S	N.I.	U	Comments
The Bed Bath				
Bring necessary equipment to the bedside and place patient flat in bed with one pillow under her head				
Remove top bed linens and cover the patient with a bath blanket; care for linens appropriately				
Move the patient to the side of the bed near you				
Wash, rinse, and dry each body part well and in a logical and convenient order				
Fold the washcloth like a mitt or in such a way that there are no loose ends				
Use washcloth wet enough to wash, lather, and rinse well but not so wet that it drips water				
Do not leave the bar of soap in the water				
Use gentle but firm, long strokes when washing, rinsing, and drying the patient				
Pay particular attention to areas where skin surfaces touch each other				
Change bath water as recommended and also if it becomes too soapy or cool				
Soak the patient's hands in the bath water as part of the bathing procedure				
Protect bed linens as necessary while bathing various body parts				

(continued)

Recommended Technique	S	N.I.	U	Comments
Use modifications of the bed-bath procedure and as indicated appropriately				
Oral Hygiene: Self-Help Patient				
Provide the necessary equipment and supplies so that the patient may brush and floss his teeth				
Oral Hygiene: Helpless Patient				
Place patient on his side with his head slightly lowered				
Clean and rinse the mouth, lips, and teeth appropriately and floss the teeth as indicated				
Use suction as indicated to prevent the patient from aspirating				
Lubricate the mouth and lips as indicated				
Care of Dentures				
Assist the patient to remove and replace dentures as necessary				
Care for the dentures over a basin of water or soft surface				
Scrub and rinse all surfaces of the dentures thoroughly with appropriate equipment				
Store dentures safely and appropriately when they are not being worn				
Nail and Hair Care				
Groom and clean the fingernails and, if ordered, the toenails with gentleness				
Use appropriate equipment and avoid injuring the patient when caring for the nails				
Protect the pillow before caring for the hair				
Arrange the hair with a proper comb and brush; braid the hair if necessary				
See to it that the patient's brush and comb are kept clean				
Shampoo the patient's hair properly, using procedures and equipment recommended by the health agency				

Recommended Technique	S	N.I.	U	Comments
Perineal Care: Self-Help Patient				
Provide the patient with proper equipment and supplies for self-care of the perineal area				
See to it that the patient's privacy is protected while he gives himself care				
Perineal Care: Helpless Patient				
Place the patient on a bedpan, or protect the bed linens properly when a bedpan is not used				
Wear gloves for the procedure or handle supplies with a forceps				
Use cotton balls, soap solution, and clear water; thoroughly scrub and rinse the area				
Clean the anal area after turning the patient to his side				
Be careful to clean the area well at the foreskin and between the labia				
Dry the patient; use protective lotion or powder as indicated				

CHAPTER 17

Comfort, Rest, and Sleep

SUMMARY

Modifying the patient's environment to promote comfort while providing sufficient sensory stimulation and privacy is a major nursing concern. The term environment, as it is used here, refers to the room where the patient receives care and the furnishings within it. When the environment is clean, safe, comfortable, and attractive, it can contribute to a sense of well being and promote rest and recovery. However, no matter how pleasant and comfortable the physical environment or how attractive and homelike the furnishings, recuperation may not occur if the patient is unable to rest or sleep.

The need for relief of sleeplessness is among the most common problems patients present. While certain drug therapy may often be indicated, its use does not eliminate the need for high-quality nursing care. Nursing measures for these patients should include actions to promote relaxation and sleep. These measures, accompanied by a description of the characteristics of relaxation and sleep, are presented in this chapter.

MATCHING QUESTIONS

Directions: For items 1 through 6, match the descriptions in Part B with the techniques in Part A.

Part A

1. _____ Effleurage
2. _____ Pítressage
3. _____ Frôlement
4. _____ Tapotement
5. _____ Vibration
6. _____ Friction

Part B
a. To brush
b. To set in motion
c. To tap
d. To knead
e. To rub
f. To skim the surface

Directions: For items 7 through 11, match the characteristics in Part B with the stages of sleep in Part A.

Part A

7. _____ Stage 1 NREM
8. _____ Stage 2 NREM
9. _____ Stage 3 NREM
10. _____ Stage 4 NREM
11. _____ REM

Part B
a. Deep sleep; parasomnias occur
b. Vivid, colorful, emotional dreams; very difficult to awaken; pauses in breathing for 15 to 20 seconds
c. Light sleep; easily aroused
d. Early phase of deep sleep; relaxed, no physical movement; difficult to arouse
e. Deep relaxation; can be awakened with effort

MULTIPLE CHOICE QUESTIONS

Directions: For items 1 through 20, circle the letter that corresponds to the best answer for each question.

1. In order for sleep to occur, which of the following is necessary:
   a. The person must be tired
   b. The person must be in a relaxed state
   c. The person must be in a recumbent position
   d. The person must be in comfortable clothing

2. Phenomena that occur every 24 hours are called:
    a. Biorhythms
    b. Ultradian rhythms
    c. Infradian rhythms
    d. Circadian rhythms

3. Sleep is characterized by:
    a. A state of drowsiness and decreased activity
    b. A state of decreased activity and mental stimulation
    c. A state of arousable unconsciousness
    d. A state of emotional rest and excessive sleepiness

4. In which stage of sleep do dreams most often occur:
    a. REM sleep
    b. Stage 2 NREM sleep
    c. Stage 3 NREM sleep
    d. Stage 4 NREM sleep

5. When an individual with insomnia cannot fall asleep within 20 minutes after getting into bed at night, it would be best to:
    a. Stay in bed and concentrate on going to sleep
    b. Stay in bed another 20 minutes and then take a sleeping pill
    c. Not worry about the situation and sleep longer in the morning
    d. Get out of bed and do something else quiet, like reading

6. Of the following colors, which promotes feelings of coolness and relaxation:
    a. Blue and brown
    b. Green and brown
    c. Blue and green
    d. Orange and green

7. Select the room temperature range that is comfortable for most people:
    a. 16° to 21° C (60° to 70° F)
    b. 18° to 24° C (65° to 75° F)
    c. 20° to 23° C (68° to 74° F)
    d. 21° to 25° C (70° to 78° F)

8. All of the following are true about the rapid eye movement phase of sleep except:
    a. It is also called paradoxical sleep because EEG waves are similar to those during wakefulness
    b. It is the lightest stage of sleep
    c. It is a period of active sleep
    d. Eye movements during this phase of sleep are energetic

9. Sleepwalking and bed-wetting usually occur during which stage or phase of sleep:
    a. Stage 4 NREM sleep
    b. Stage 3 NREM Sleep
    c. Stage 2 NREM sleep
    d. REM sleep

10. Secretion of the hormone melatonin is triggered by:
    a. Activity
    b. Bright light
    c. Darkness
    d. The environment

11. The term photoperiod refers to:
    a. A technique for stimulating light receptors in the eye
    b. A technique for inducing sleep for persons with insomnia
    c. The number of times light therapy can be used effectively
    d. The number of daylight hours to which a person is accustomed

12. Seasonal affective disorder occurs during:
    a. The fall
    b. The winter
    c. The spring
    d. The summer

13. The best sources of L-tryptophan are:
    a. Protein foods and dairy products
    b. Shellfish and vegetables
    c. Dairy products and fruits
    d. Protein foods and chocolate

14. Narcolepsy is a condition characterized by:
    a. Excessive anxiety
    b. Excessive sleeping
    c. Excessive fatigue
    d. Excessive sleepiness

15. It is appropriate for a newborn to sleep:
    a. 16 to 20 hours per 24-hour period
    b. 10 to 16 hours in addition to two or three naps
    c. 10 to 12 hours in addition to one or two naps
    d. 8 to 10 hours in addition to one nap or rest period

16. Five-and six-year-olds spend which of the following percentages in REM sleep:
    a. 50%
    b. 35%
    c. 25%
    d. 20%

17. In severe cases of sleep apnea, which of the following techniques are recommended:
    a. Suggest the individual wear a sleep collar at night
    b. Awaken the individual to restore breathing
    c. Give the individual carbon dioxide before bedtime
    d. Suggest the individual wear a special breathing mask at night

18. Parasomnias are best described as:
    a. Bedtime rituals
    b. Relaxation techniques
    c. Therapeutic use of exercises for sleep
    d. Activities that occur during sleep

19. Nocturnal myoclonus is synonymous with:
    a. Restless leg syndrome
    b. Sleepwalking
    c. Hypopnea syndrome
    d. Bedwetting

20. All of the following are characteristics of the sundown syndrome except:
    a. Alert and oriented in the evening
    b. Disorganized thinking
    c. Restlessness
    d. Wandering about

TRUE OR FALSE QUESTIONS

Directions: For items 1 through 10, decide if the statement is true or false and mark T or F in the space provided.

1. _____   During sleep, individuals pass back and forth through the phases and stages of sleep.
2. _____   Snoring occurs during stage 3 NREM sleep.
3. _____   During REM sleep, 15-to 20-second pauses in breathing are normal.
4. _____   Based on current research, REM sleep always precedes NREM sleep.
5. _____   Shift workers have little difficulty adjusting their sleep-wake cycles because indoor lighting is sufficient to suppress melatonin.
6. _____   The term phototherapy refers to a technique for suppressing melatonin by stimulating light receptors in the eye.
7. _____   Symptoms associated with seasonal affective disorder spontaneously disappear as the amount of daylight increases.
8. _____   L-tryptophan is known to facilitate sleep.
9. _____   Tranquilizers are drugs that induce sleep.
10. _____   The incidence of sleep apnea is highest among middle-aged women who snore.

SHORT ANSWER QUESTIONS

Directions: Read each of the following statements and supply the word(s) necessary in the space provided.

1. List four of the components of phototherapy used to relieve the symptoms of seasonal affective disorder as discussed in this chapter.
    a. _____
    b. _____
    c. _____
    d. _____

2. Identify five tips for patient teaching to promote sleep.
    a. _____
    b. _____
    c. _____
    d. _____
    e. _____

3. State five tips for patient teaching related to facilitating the use of progressive relaxation.
    a. _____
    b. _____
    c. _____
    d. _____
    e. _____

CRITICAL THINKING EXERCISES

1. Recall an occasion when your sleep was disturbed and you were unable to get as much sleep as you generally need. How did this affect your productivity, ability to concentrate on necessary tasks, relationships, and mood? Draw on this experience to understand how clients with sleep alterations are handicapped.

   Discuss measures nurses can take to promote rest and sleep. Use this experience to project the effect of chronic sleep deprivation on your professional practice.

2. Visit a residential care setting and use observation and interview techniques to identify factors that are compromising the rest and sleep of the residents. Strategize about how the environment and nursing care could be modified to minimize these factors.

3. Describe adjustments you make when promoting rest and sleep in special situations:
   a. When the patient is an infant or child

   b. When the patient is elderly

4. Prepare a teaching plan for each of the following topics:

Topic for Teaching	Points to Cover in a Teaching Program
Sleep and its role in well being including amount required by age groups.	
Drug use in relation to drugs used to promote sleep.	

PERFORMANCE CHECKLIST

A. This section allows you to examine your practice of safety measures and your techniques for maintaining the patient's environment.

1. Place a check mark in the "S" ("satisfactory") column if you used the recommended technique.
2. Place a check mark in the "N.I." ("needs improvement") column if you used some but not all of each recommended technique.
3. Place a check mark in the "U" ("unsatisfactory") column if you forgot to include that particular recommended technique.
4. The section for comment allows space to make notes about when further practice is indicated, what errors you made, suggestions that will improve your skills, and so on.

Recommended Technique	S	N.I.	U	Comments
The Room				
Has attractive and practical floor and wall coverings and wall accessories				
Provides good lighting for the patient and for health workers				
Has provisions for regulating temperature, humidity, and ventilation				
Has features so that the patient can be assured of privacy				
Has an adjustable bed with an overbed table				
Has several pillows and has a mattress that is sufficiently firm to provide good body alignment				
Has chairs that are comfortable and convenient for the patient and visitors				
Has personal care items and a bedside stand available				
Has diversional items, such as a television, radio, and telephone				
To Provide Privacy				
Use cubicle drapes and screens appropriately				
Close room door when giving care				
Drape patient carefully when giving care				

(continued)

Recommended Technique	S	N.I.	U	Comments
Provide privacy when the patient uses a bedpan or urinal				
Knock before entering a door				
Help visitors find the patient they wish to visit				
To Control Noise				
Handle equipment as quietly as possible. Handle dinnerware and trays quietly				
Answer telephone promptly and speak in a normal tone of voice				
Avoid calling down corridors				
Avoid laughing and chatting in corridors and lounges				
Limit reporting to the nurses' station and conference rooms				
Help keep television sets and radios at a low volume				
To Control Odors				
Discard waste and refuse promptly				
Empty bedpans, urinals, and emesis basins promptly				
Remove leftover food from rooms promptly				
Use personal grooming measures for yourself and for patients to prevent unpleasant odors				

B. Examine your techniques when stripping and making an unoccupied bed and complete the following form.

Recommended Technique	S	N.I.	U	Comments
Bring hamper to the bedside				
Avoid touching uniform with soiled linens and avoid shaking linens during the procedure				
Bring necessary linens to the bedside and arrange them in order of their use on clean furniture				
Place the bed in the high position and drop bed siderails				
Loosen linens while moving around the bed				
Roll all soiled linens snugly in the bottom sheet and place them directly into the hamper				

Recommended Technique	S	N.I.	U	Comments
Place bottom linens on the bed, one piece at a time, and unfold them in place after centering them				
Secure bottom linens in place				
Center and unfold top linens on the bed; secure them well but allow for toe room				
Cover pillows in place and position them properly on the bed				
Place the signal device so that it is conveniently located for the patient				
Examine your technique when assisting the patient with a sleep disturbance				
Know the patient's diagnosis and her usual patterns of sleep				
Provide for an environment that promotes sleep				
Allow the patient to observe her usual bedtime habits to the greatest extent possible				
Remove causes, such as pain, for restlessness and sleeplessness and use techniques to help the patient relax				
Take steps to avoid waking a sleeping patient				
Use prescribed medications for restlessness and sleeplessness judiciously				
Consult others for assistance with the care of the restless and sleepless patient as necessary				
Record techniques you have found helpful when assisting the restless and sleepless patient				

C H A P T E R   1 8

Safety

SUMMARY

No age group is immune to accidental injury. However, there are distinct differences among various age groups that contribute to their risks and to the type of accident or injury that may occur. These differences are highlighted in this chapter. The appropriate steps to be taken when fires, accidents, or injuries occur are suggested so that students may familiarize themselves with nursing responsibilities surrounding these incidents.

MATCHING QUESTIONS

Directions: For items 1 through 10, match the definitions in Part B with the terms in Part A.

Part A

1. _____ Hazards
2. _____ Burns
3. _____ Asphyxiation
4. _____ Drowning
5. _____ Macroshock
6. _____ Poisoning
7. __C__ Restraint
8. _____ Microshock
9. _____ Ground
10. _____ Safety

Part B

a. Measures that prevent unintentional injuries
b. Distribution of low-amperage electricity over a large body area
c. A device that restricts movement
d. Diverts electrical energy to earth
e. A type of skin injury from chemicals
f. Ingestion or inhalation of a toxic substance
g. Distribution of low-voltage, high-amperage electricity over a large body area
h. Inability to breathe
i. Fluid interferes with ventilation
j. Potentially dangerous conditions in the physical surroundings

MULTIPLE CHOICE QUESTIONS

Directions: For items 1 through 12, circle the letter that corresponds to the best answer for each question.

1. The content of a Class B fire extinguisher is:
   a. Water under pressure
   b. Carbon dioxide
   c. Dry chemicals
   d. Graphite

2. The first measure the nurse must carry out when a fire occurs is:
   a. Notify the switchboard using the proper code
   b. Turn off the oxygen supply near the fire
   c. Use the appropriate fire extinguisher
   d. Evacuate the people from the room with the fire

3. When an accident occurs, which of the following steps should be taken first:
   a. Report the accident to the proper person promptly
   b. Comfort and reassure the patient who was involved
   c. Check the condition of the involved patient
   d. Call for the assistance of other health personnel

4. When an accident occurs, which of the following steps should be taken last:
   a. Report the accident to the proper authorities
   b. Enter all of the information on an accident report
   c. Notify the physician that her patient has had an accident
   d. Comfort and reassure the patient involved

5. A thermal burn is a skin injury caused by:
   a. Heat
   b. Lightning
   c. Steam
   d. Electricity

6. The term asphyxiation means:
   a. The inability to breathe
   b. Fluid in the airway
   c. Discharge of electricity through the body
   d. Inhalation of a toxic substance

7. The body is susceptible to electrical shock because:
   a. It is well insulated
   b. It is grounded
   c. It acts as a resistor
   d. It is a good conductor

8. The most prevalent type of accident experienced by older adults is:
   a. Poisoning
   b. Falls
   c. Burns
   d. Asphyxiation

9. Which of the following acronyms incorporate the steps found in most fire plans:
   a. ABC
   b. OBRA
   c. NFPA
   d. RACE

10. Macroshock is best described as:
    a. The distribution of low-amperage electricity over a large body area
    b. The distribution of high-amperage electricity over a large body area
    c. A fatal electrical current delivered directly to the heart
    d. Resistance to the movement of electric current offered by intact skin

11. Class A fire extinguishers are used for fires involving:
    a. Flammable liquid
    b. Electricity
    c. Paper or wood
    d. Any type of fire

12. Risks associated with the use of physical restraints include:
    a. Constipation, incontinence, infection
    b. Falls, confusion, asphyxiation
    c. Dementia, disorientation, disability
    d. Visual impairment, hypotension, urinary urgency

TRUE OR FALSE QUESTIONS

Directions: For items 1 through 10, decide if the statement is true or false and mark T or F in the space provided.

1. __F__ One of the general reasons to use restraints is to provide for as much movement as possible within the restraint.

2. _____ In the event of a fire, it is best to place bath blankets at the threshold of doors where smoke is leaking.

3. _____ Smoke is sometimes more deadly than the fire with which it is associated.

4. _____ Carbon monoxide can be present in the absence of smoke.

5. _____ Victims of warm-water drownings are more likely to be resuscitated than those who drown in cold water.

6. _____ Poisonings never occur in health care institutions.

7. _____ Educating children is the only way to prevent childhood poisoning in the home.

8. __F__ Falls may be prevented by determining which patients are at risk.

9. __F__ Restrained patients are eight times more likely to die during hospitalization than patients who are not restrained.

10. __F__ Among older adults who fall, 90% are eventually transferred to a nursing home.

33%

SHORT ANSWER QUESTIONS

Directions: Read each of the following statements and supply the word(s) necessary in the space provided.

1. State (briefly) why it is necessary to obtain a physician's written order before restraining a patient. _____

2. List three methods to help prevent falls as suggested in this chapter.
   a. __lighted room__
   b. __use cane__
   c. __remove clutter__

3. List the risk factors suggested in this chapter for accidental falls. _____

4. List the seven steps the nurse should follow when a fire occurs.
   a. _____
   b. _____
   c. _____
   d. _____
   e. _____

f. _____

g. _____

5. List the six steps the nurse should follow when using a fire extinguisher.

a. _____

b. _____

c. _____

d. _____

e. _____

f. _____

CRITICAL THINKING EXERCISES:

1. Describe adjustments necessary to provide a safe and comfortable environment:

a. When the patient is an infant or child

b. When the patient is helpless

c. When the patient is elderly

2. Identify nursing strategies that would be likely to secure client cooperation in making these changes.

PERFORMANCE CHECKLIST

A. This section allows you to examine your techniques for maintaining safety in the patient's environment.
1. Place a check mark in the "S" ("satisfactory") column if you used the recommended technique.
2. Place a check mark in the "N.I." ("needs improvement") column if you used some but not all of each recommended technique.
3. Place a check mark in the "U" ("unsatisfactory") column if you forgot to include that particular recommended technique.
4. The section for comment allows space to make notes about when further practice is indicated, what errors you made, suggestions that will improve your skills, and so on.

Recommended Technique	S	N.I.	U	Comments
To Use Restraints				
Obtain a physician's order as soon as possible				
Explain to the patient and family why restraints are to be used				
Allow some mobility and do not apply restraints too tightly				
Avoid applying restraints over bony prominences				
Position the patient comfortably before applying restraints				
Keep the patient in sight whenever restraints are used				
Apply restraints to parts of the body correctly and safely				
Fasten restraints to the bed's frame, not the siderails				
Give appropriate nursing care to the restrained patient				
To Prevent Falls				
Place bed in a low position for the ambulatory patient				
Use nonskid mats or strips in tubs and showers				
Use tub and shower stools and handrails appropriately				

(continued)

Recommended Technique	S	N.I.	U	Comments
Use equipment and supplies only for their intended purposes				
Have patients use good walking shoes when ambulating				
Do not allow litter to gather on floors and in corridors				
Have patients in wheelchairs use wide doorways, ramps, and elevators				
See to it that spilled liquids are wiped up promptly				
To Prevent Electrical Injuries				
Use plugs and outlets with grounds whenever possible				
Remove plugs from wall sockets by grasping the plugs				
Use electrical equipment for its intended purpose only				
See to it that electrical equipment is in good working order				
Keep electrical equipment away from bathtubs, sinks, and showers				
Avoid wearing wet shoes or standing in water when using equipment				
Do not kink electrical cords or use frayed cords				
To Prevent Fires				
Know where emergency exits and fire extinguishers are				
Use appropriate precautions when oxygen is in use				
Help enforce smoking regulations				
Observe patients for safety when they smoke				
Avoid storing materials that may lead to spontaneous combustion				
To Prevent Poisoning				
Know where emergency instructions are posted				
Help see to it that poisonous substances are conspicuously labeled				

Recommended Technique	S	N.I.	U	Comments
Store poisonous substances properly				
Do not place poisonous substances in another container				
See to it that medications are stored securely and properly				
To Prevent Scalds and Burns				
Check the temperature of bath and shower water				
Agitate water when adding hot water to a tub				
Use heating pads according to agency policy				
To Prevent Drowning and Asphyxiation				
Offer small bits of food to patients while helping them to eat				
Offer liquids to helpless patients with care				
Do not leave a patient alone in a tub or shower if they are weak or cognitively impaired				
Never leave a child alone in a tub, shower, or bathroom				
Miscellaneous				
Observe practices of medical and surgical asepsis				
See to it that the patient's call device is always handy for use				

B. Examine your techniques, or those of another nurse, when an accident occurs and complete the following form.

Recommended Technique	S	N.I.	U	Comments
Check the patient's condition immediately				
Call for assistance				
Do not move the patient until it is safe to do so				
Comfort and reassure the patient appropriately				
Offer no explanations until after consulting a supervisor				
Notify proper personnel of the accident				
Document the accident properly, including preparing an incident report				

CHAPTER 19

Pain Management

SUMMARY

Pain is an unpleasant sensation usually associated with disease or injury. It also has an emotional aspect referred to as suffering. Research shows that the pain experience is highly subjective and individualized. Pain exists when and to what extent the patient says it does.

Pain is probably the major cause of physical distress among patients. This chapter provides information about pain and techniques for pain relief.

MATCHING QUESTIONS

Directions: For items 1 through 5, match the descriptions in Part B with the standards in Part A.

Part A
1. _____ Standard I
2. _____ Standard II
3. _____ Standard III
4. _____ Standard IV
5. _____ Standard V

Part B
a. Adherence to standards is monitored by an interdisciplinary committee
b. Patients are informed verbally and in writing that pain relief is important
c. Acute pain and cancer pain are recognized and effectively treated
d. Information about analgesics is readily available
e. Explicit policies for use of advanced analgesic technologies are defined

Directions: For items 6 through 10, match the descriptions in Part B with the types of pain in Part A.

Part A
6. _____ Cutaneous
7. _____ Visceral
8. _____ Neuropathic
9. _____ Referred
10. _____ Phantom

Part B
a. Pain with atypical characteristics
b. Discomfort perceived away from the site of stimulation
c. Discomfort arising from internal organs
d. Deep pain in tissues that have been surgically removed
e. Discomfort that originates at the skin level

MULTIPLE CHOICE QUESTIONS

Directions: For items 1 through 10, circle the letter that corresponds to the best answer for each question.

1. Which of the following statements most accurately describes a characteristic of pain:
   a. Pain is objective in nature
   b. Responses to pain vary widely
   c. Pain is always associated with bodily damage
   d. Pain is not a demanding situation

2. Acute pain is best described as:
   a. Physical discomfort that exists less than six months
   b. Physical discomfort that usually lasts longer than six months
   c. Physical discomfort that usually lasts longer than two months
   d. Physical discomfort that usually lasts less than two months

3. Of the following statements, which best defines referred pain:
   a. Physical discomfort that exists less than six months
   b. Physical discomfort that exists in the part of the body that is injured
   c. Pain in an area of the body that results from some mental or emotional origin
   d. Pain in an area of the body that is some distance from the part that is injured

4. Acupuncture and acupressure may stimulate the production of which of the following chemicals to relieve pain:
   a. Morphine
   b. Endorphins
   c. Insulin
   d. Adrenaline

5. Biofeedback is best described as:
   a. A training program that helps the individual by substituting for his drug therapy
   b. A training program that produces a subconscious condition that is used to control pain
   c. A training program that helps the individual become aware of certain body changes
   d. A program used to produce simple pressure on various body parts to help reduce pain

6. The patient's discomfort is most likely relieved by a placebo in which of the following situations:
   a. When the discomfort is only mild
   b. When the discomfort is imagined or anticipated
   c. When the patient is almost recovered
   d. When the patient has confidence in his caregivers

7. One of the advantages for using transcutaneous electrical nerve stimulation (TENS) is:
   a. It can be used for pregnant women
   b. It can only be used intermittently
   c. It is nonnarcotic without toxic effects
   d. It requires no training in its use

8. A parenteral dose of 10 mg of morphine sulfate given every 3 to 4 hours is equal to which of the following dosages of the same drug given orally?
   a. 7.5 mg by mouth every 3 to 4 hours
   b. 30 mg by mouth every 3 to 4 hours
   c. 150 mg by mouth every 3 to 4 hours
   d. 300 mg by mouth every 2 to 3 hours

9. An equianalgesic dose of a medication refers to:
   a. The amount required to provide a favorable response over time
   b. The amount associated with sympathetic nervous system responses
   c. An unpleasant sensation associated with the adjusted oral dose over time
   d. The adjusted oral dose that provides the same relief as a parenteral dose

10. Nondrug interventions for pain relief are most likely to be used for which of the following types of pain?
    a. Acute pain
    b. Chronic pain
    c. Visceral pain
    d. Cutaneous pain

TRUE OR FALSE QUESTIONS

Directions: For items 1 through 12, decide if the statement is true or false and mark T or F in the space provided.

1. _____ Pain threshold is the ability of an individual to endure pain.

2. _____ Discomfort in a location distant from the diseased or injured part of the body is known as phantom limb pain.

3. _____ The point at which the sensation of pain becomes noticeable appears to be about the same among healthy persons.

4. _____ Individuals from different cultures tolerate pain in the same manner.

5. _____ Anxiety and fear are common emotions accompanying pain.

6. _____ The human body is able to adapt to the sensation of pain.

7. _____ When the patient is allowed to help select methods to relieve his pain, he usually has better results.

8. _____ Patient-controlled analgesia is used primarily in hospitals for patients with chronic pain.

9. _____ The initial dose administered through a patient-controlled analgesia system is the same as the amount released each time the patient activates the system.

10. _____ The TENS unit is contraindicated in pregnancy because its effect is unknown.

11. _____ Addiction is a pattern of compulsive drug use accompanied by a continued craving for the drug and a need to use the drug for effects other than pain relief.

12. _____ Hypnosis is a trancelike state during which perception and memory are altered.

SHORT ANSWER QUESTIONS

1. List eight of the advantages of using patient-controlled analgesia suggested in this chapter.

   a. _____

   b. _____

   c. _____

   d. _____

   e. _____

   f. _____

   g. _____

   h. _____

2. Identify five components of pain assessment as suggested in this chapter.

   a. _____

   b. _____

   c. _____

   d. _____

   e. _____

CRITICAL THINKING EXERCISES

1. Plan a teaching program for a woman in labor and complete the following form.

Topic for Teaching	Points to Cover in a Teaching Program
Pain and its role in the labor process	
Measures to control pain	

2. Read the following case study and use your nursing process skills to prepare a nursing care plan related to pain management for this patient.

A 24-month-old infant with AIDS is hospitalized with infectious diarrhea. She is well known to the pediatric staff, and there is real concern that she might not pull through this admission. She has suffered many of the complications of AIDS and is no stranger to pain. At the present time, the skin on her buttocks is raw and excoriated, and tears stream down her face whenever she is moved. Her blood pressure also shoots up when she is touched. The severity of her illness has left her extremely weak and listless, and her foster mother reports that she no longer recognizes her child. When alone in her crib, she seldom moves, and moans softly. Several nurses have expressed great frustration caring for her because they find it hard to perform even simple nursing measures like turning, diapering and weighing her when they see how much pain these procedures cause.

From: Taylor C., Lillis C. & Lemone P. (1997). *Study guide to accompany fundamentals of nursing: The art and science of nursing care. (p. 243)*. Philadelphia: Lippincott.

PERFORMANCE CHECKLIST

A. This section allows you to examine your techniques for assisting the patient with pain control.

1. Place a check mark in the "S" ("satisfactory") column if you used the recommended technique.
2. Place a check mark in the "N.I." ("needs improvement") column if you used some but not all of each recommended technique.
3. Place a check mark in the "U" ("unsatisfactory") column if you forgot to include that particular recommended technique.
4. The section for comment allows space to make notes about when further practice is indicated, what errors you made, suggestions that will improve your skills, and so on.

Recommended Technique	S	N.I.	U	Comments
Know the patient's diagnosis, his plan of therapy, and his usual responses to pain				
Determine the nature of the patient's pain accurately				
Observe the patient in pain regularly and note any signs/symptoms that accompany his pain				
Take appropriate steps to decrease or remove the cause of the patient's pain as indicated				
Use various techniques to help a patient relax and obtain relief from pain				
Remain with the patient in pain and listen if the patient wishes to talk about his pain				
Use prescribed medications for pain as ordered				
Consult others for assistance with the care of the patient in pain as necessary				
Record techniques you have found helpful when assisting the patient in pain				

CHAPTER 20

Oxygenation

SUMMARY

Oxygen is essential for almost every form of animal and plant life. It is used by each cell of the human body to metabolize nutrients and produce energy. This chapter presents information on the bedside procedure for measuring oxygen content of the blood, the types of oxygen equipment used in oxygen therapy, and the skills needed to maintain respiratory function. Tips for physical assessment of the patient receiving oxygen therapy are also presented.

MATCHING QUESTIONS

Directions: For items 1 through 10, match the definition in Part B with the term in Part A.

Part A
1. _____ External respiration
2. _____ Ventilation
3. _____ Respiration
4. _____ Internal respiration
5. _____ Hypoxemia
6. _____ Oxygen saturation
7. _____ Deep breathing
8. _____ Incentive spirometry
9. _____ Pursed-lip spirometry
10. _____ Hypoxia

Part B
a. Transfer of oxygen across cellular membranes
b. Inadequate oxygen at the cellular level
c. A technique for maximizing ventilation
d. Transfer of oxygen from alveoli to blood
e. Movement of air in and out of the lungs
f. Controlled ventilation in which expiration is prolonged
g. The percent of oxygen bound to hemoglobin

h. Mechanism by which oxygen is delivered to the cells
i. A technique for measuring volume of air inhaled
j. Insufficient oxygen within arterial blood

Directions: For items 11 through 14, match the characteristics in Part B with the types of masks in Part A.

Part A
11. _____ Simple mask
12. _____ Partial rebreather mask
13. _____ Non-rebreather mask
14. _____ Venti mask

Part B
a. All exhaled air leaves mask
b. Has large, ringed tube and dial system for specific amount of oxygen
c. Attached to reservoir bag; one third exhaled air enters bag
d. Fits over nose and mouth

MULTIPLE CHOICE QUESTIONS

Directions: For items 1 through 10, circle the letter that corresponds to the best answer for each question.

1. The patient's response to oxygen therapy is most accurately determined by:
   a. Examinations of the arterial blood gases
   b. Changes in the color of his skin and nailbeds
   c. Changes in his vital signs
   d. Changes in his level of consciousness

2. One of the earliest signs of oxygen toxicity is:
   a. A productive cough
   b. A dry cough
   c. Loss of consciousness
   d. Flushing of the skin

3. To crack an oxygen tank means to:
   a. Stabilize the tank on a stand
   b. Attach a humidifier to the tank
   c. Regulate the flow meter of the tank
   d. Clean the tank's outlet of debris

4. For patients with chronic lung conditions, oxygen via nasal cannula is usually prescribed at:
   a. 2 to 3 liters per minute
   b. 2 to 4 liters per minute
   c. 3 to 6 liters per minute
   d. 4 to 7 liters per minute

5. For a patient with a chronic lung condition, high levels of oxygen may decrease or even stop respirations because:
   a. His body is not accustomed to breathing correctly
   b. The oxygen level in the body will go too high
   c. His body is accustomed to higher than normal carbon dioxide levels
   d. His body is accustomed to lower than normal carbon dioxide levels

6. The Venturi mask delivers a supply of up to:
   a. 10% oxygen
   b. 20% oxygen
   c. 30% oxygen
   d. 40% oxygen

7. Lung collapse is primarily caused by:
   a. The loss of negative pressure within the pleural space
   b. The loss of negative pressure within the lungs
   c. The loss of positive pressure within the pleural space
   d. The loss of fluid pressure within the pleural cavity

8. The water seal chest drainage system is designed to prevent:
   a. Negative pressure from reentering the lungs
   b. Negative pressure from reentering the pleural cavity
   c. Atmospheric air from reentering the lungs
   d. Atmospheric air from reentering the pleural space

9. Patients receiving oxygen via the transtracheal method usually achieve adequate oxygenation with:
   a. More oxygen flow than other methods
   b. Less oxygen flow than other methods
   c. The same amount of oxygen flow as other methods
   d. The method used does not affect the amount of oxygen used

10. Oxygen delivered at 4L per minute for a period of time is humidified because:
    a. It is a means of decreasing the amount of oxygen used
    b. The addition of water can deliver the exact amount of oxygen required
    c. Oxygen is very drying to mucous membranes
    d. Oxygen has a bad taste if it is not humidified

TRUE OF FALSE QUESTIONS

Directions: For items 1 through 10, decide if the statement is true or false and mark T or F in the space provided.

1. _____ Hypoxemia is defined as a deficiency in the amount of oxygen in inspired air.

2. _____ Oxygen is a flammable gas.

3. _____ Oxygen is usually administered via cannula for patients suffering with smoke inhalation or carbon monoxide poisoning.

4. _____ Lung collapse is due to the loss of positive pressure within the pleural space.

5. _____ There are no lung sounds heard over the areas in which the lung has deflated.

6. _____ A water-seal drainage system should be emptied routinely.

7. _____ Failure of the water to fluctuate within the water-seal drainage system may mean that the patient's lung has expanded.

8. _____ A major advantage of the nasal cannula is that it allows 10 or more liters of oxygen to be administered without causing drying of the mucous membranes.

9. _____ High percentages of oxygen via nasal cannula are needed by patients with chronic lung diseases.

10. _____ Since transtracheal catheters are made of plastic, they can be cleaned and reused.

SHORT ANSWER QUESTIONS

Directions: Read each of the following statements and supply the word(s) necessary in the space provided.

1. Identify the nursing guidelines for the safe use of oxygen as suggested in this chapter.
   a. _____
   b. _____
   c. _____
   d. _____

e. _____

f. _____

g. _____

2. Identify five common signs of inadequate oxygenation.

a. _____

b. _____

c. _____

d. _____

e. _____

3. List seven components that are part of the evaluation of the effectiveness of oxygen administration.

a. _____

b. _____

c. _____

d. _____

e. _____

f. _____

g. _____

4. List four suggested actions that should be taken when using oxygen dispensed from a tank.

a. _____

b. _____

c. _____

d. _____

5. List five methods of administering oxygen.

a. _____

b. _____

c. _____

d. _____

e. _____

CRITICAL THINKING EXERCISE

Arrange with your clinical instructor to spend some time observing the respiratory therapist administer various types of respiratory treatments. Describe each including the purpose/goal, kinds of patients treated and results. Identify nursing activities appropriate for effective patient care and coordination of these activities. Determine when/how you might need to be the patients' advocate when they are receiving respiratory therapy.

PERFORMANCE CHECKLIST

A. This section allows you to examine your techniques for assisting a patient receiving oxygen therapy.
  1. Place a check mark in the "S" ("satisfactory") column if you used the recommended technique.
  2. Place a check mark in the "N.I." ("needs improvement") column if you used some but not all of each recommended technique.

3. Place a check mark in the "U" (unsatisfactory") column if you forgot to include that particular recommended technique.
4. The section for comment allows space to make notes about when further practice is indicated, what errors you made, suggestions that will improve your skills, and so on.

Recommended Technique	S	N.I.	U	Comments
Note that humidified oxygen is being delivered to the device for giving oxygen before putting it on the patient				
Place a cannula into the patient's nostrils, using padding if necessary, so that skin irritation is avoided				
Place a lubricated catheter properly into a nostril a distance about equal to the distance from nostril to earlobe				
Check the placement of a catheter in the oropharynx and secure it to the nose				
Place a mask over the face, secure it in place				
Change a disposable cannula, catheter, or mask, or clean a reusable one, at least every 8 hours; more often if indicated				
Check at regular intervals that the patient is receiving humidified oxygen at the prescribed rate				
Observe the patient for oxygen toxicity				
Check the supply of oxygen at regular intervals and know the agency policy for obtaining additional oxygen				
Check at regular intervals that the cannula, catheter, or mask is not irritating the patient's skin				

(continued)

Recommended Technique	S	N.I.	U	Comments
Take appropriate steps when the device is irritating the skin or mucous membranes				
Offer the patient oral hygiene at regular and frequent intervals				
Observe precautions at all times for the safe delivery of oxygen				
Post "No Smoking" signs				
Note that electrical equipment is in good working order				
Avoid petroleum and acetone products				
Check to see that oil and grease are not used near oxygen equipment				
See to it that there are no open flames in the presence of oxygen				
See to it that fire extinguishers are handy and know how to use them				
If oxygen is in a tank, see to it that the tank is secured properly on its stand				
Avoid wearing clothing that produces static electricity when around oxygen				

B. Examine your techniques for maintaining water-seal drainage and complete the following form.

Recommended Technique	S	N.I.	U	Comments
Review patient's medical record to determine the condition that necessitated the chest tube insertion				
Determine if there are one or two chest tubes and note date of insertion				
Check medical orders to determine if drainage is being collected gravity by or with suction				
Perform physical assessment as soon after report as possible				
Take a roll of tape and a container of distilled water with you				
Introduce yourself; explain purpose of interaction; wash your hands				
Check to see that hemostats are at bedside				

Recommended Technique	S	N.I.	U	Comments
Turn off suction regulator; assess patient's lung sounds				
Inspect the dressing for signs of soiling or looseness				
Palpate the skin around the insertion site to feel for and listen for air crackling in the tissue				
Inspect all connections; reinforce loose ones with tape				
Make sure tubing is unkinked and hangs freely into drainage system				
Make sure fluid level in water-seal chamber is at 2-cm level				
Add distilled water to mark if the fluid level is low				
Note if water is rising and falling with each respiration				
Observe for continuous bubbling in the water-seal chamber				
Correct for continuous bubbling as appropriate				
Maintain water level in suction chamber at 20 cm				
Regulate suction to produce gentle bubbling				
Observe nature and amount of drainage				
Keep drainage system below the chest				
Curl and secure tubing as appropriate				
Encourage coughing and deep breathing				
Instruct patient to move about in bed, ambulate, and exercise shoulder on the side with the tubing				
Never clamp tubing for long periods of time				
Mark drainage level on the collection chamber at the end of your shift				
Document assessment findings, care provided, and amount of drainage during the period of care				

PERFORMANCE CHECKLIST

This section allows you to examine your techniques for controlling the spread of microorganisms in the patient's environment.

1. Place a check mark in the "S" ("satisfactory") column if you used the recommended technique.
2. Place a check mark in the "N.I." ("needs improvement") column if you used some but not all of each recommended technique.
3. Place a check mark in the "U" ("unsatisfactory") column if you forgot to include that particular recommended technique.
4. The section for comment allows space to make notes about when further practice is indicated, what errors you made, suggestions that will improve your skills, and so on.

Recommended Technique	S	N.I.	U	Comments
Medical Asepsis When Giving Care				
Wash hands before and after giving care				
Handle all discharges correctly				
Place damp or wet items in a waterproof bag				
Discard disposable equipment according to agency policy				
Flush away contents of bedpans and urinals promptly				
Use equipment for one patient only				
Cover breaks in the skin with sterile dressings				
Prevent soiled equipment and supplies from touching your uniform				
Consider the floor heavily contaminated				
Avoid raising dust and lint				
Clean the least soiled areas first, heavily soiled areas last				
Pour liquids to be discarded directly into a drain or toilet				
Avoid spilling and splashing liquids				
Help keep the patient's room as clean, bright, dry, and airy as possible				
Do not use equipment when there is any doubt about its being clean or sterile				

(continued)

Recommended Technique	S	N.I.	U	Comments
Personal Grooming				
Keep the hair cut short or secured well if long				
Wear only plain-band rings				
Wear wristwatch high enough so that it does not become contaminated				
Do not wear loose-fitting bracelets				
Keep fingernails short and well groomed				
Follow agency policy about the use of nail polish				
Practices of Everyday Living				
Cover the nose and mouth when coughing or sneezing				
Wash hands before handling food				
Use individual personal care items				
Wash hands after using the bathroom				
Handwashing				
Stand near sink but without touching it with the uniform				
Observe agency policy about opening and closing faucets or use foot and knee controls properly				
Keep hands and forearms lower than elbows and avoid touching the sink during the entire procedure				
Use warm water and enough soap to produce a good lather on the hands and wrists				
If bar soap is used, keep bar in hands until end of washing and drop it into the dish without touching it				
Use firm, rubbing, and circular motion while cleaning the palms, backs of hands, fingers, and wrists				
Wash for recommended periods for light and heavy soilage				
Rinse and soap two to three times when soilage is especially heavy				
Finish by rinsing washed areas well under running water				

Recommended Technique	S	N.I.	U	Comments
Clean surfaces under nails with orange stick at least once a day and whenever hands are heavily soiled				
Pat dry hands and wrists				
Apply lotion to hands and wrists as necessary				
Surgical Asepsis				
Open sterile trays by folding top layer away from you and bottom layer toward you				
Touch only out side of wrapper when opening a tray				
Do not walk away from a sterile field or reach across it				
Avoid talking, coughing, or sneezing over a sterile field				
Hold sterile objects above the level of the waist				
See to it that a sterile field remains dry				
Handle sterile equipment with sterile forceps or with hands after putting on sterile gloves				
Don sterile gloves in a way so that the hands do not touch the outside surface of the gloves				
Avoid draft in the work area				
Use only sterile equipment and supplies, and replace if there is doubt about sterility				

PERFORMANCE CHECKLIST

This section allows you to examine your techniques for preventing the spread of communicable diseases.

1. Place a check mark in the "S" ("satisfactory") column if you used the recommended technique.
2. Place a check mark in the "N.I." ("needs improvement") column if you used some but not all of each recommended technique.
3. Place a check mark in the "U" ("unsatisfactory") column if you forgot to include that particular recommended technique.
4. The section for comment allows space to make notes of about when further practice is indicated, what errors you made, suggestions that will improve your skills, and so on.

Recommended Technique	S	N.I.	U	Comments
Removal of Isolation Garments				
Untie or unfasten waist ties				
Remove gloves and dispose of in the proper container				
Wash hands				
Turn the faucet off with a paper towel				
Remove the mask and discard it in the disposable trash or laundry container				
Untie or unfasten neck closure				
Remove the gown				
Discard the gown in the trash container if it is a disposable type or in the soiled linen if made of fabric				
Wash hands				
Open the isolation door with a clean paper towel, touching the doorknob only				
Discard the paper towel into the wastebasket inside the patient's room				
Leave the room taking care not to touch anything				
Go directly to the utility room and wash hands one final time				

PERFORMANCE CHECKLIST

A. This section allows you to examine your technique for assisting the patient with improving posture and body mechanics.

1. Place a check mark in the "S" ("satisfactory") column if you used the recommended technique.
2. Place a check mark in the "N.I." ("needs improvement") column if you used some but not all of each recommended technique.
3. Place a check mark in the "U" ("unsatisfactory") column if you forgot to include the particular recommended technique.
4. The section for comment allows space to make notes about when further practice is indicated, what errors you made, suggestions that will improve your skills, and so on.

Recommended Technique	S	N.I.	U	Comments
Posture When Standing				
Place feet parallel to each other, at right angles to the lower legs				
Place feet about 10 to 20 centimeters (4 to 8 inches) apart				
Distribute weight equally on both feet				
Have knees slightly bent				
Use an internal girdle and a long midriff				
Hold the head erect with the chin slightly in				
Posture When Sitting				
Place both feet on the floor, legs uncrossed				
Knees bent; popliteal area free from edge of chair				
Hold the head erect with the chin slightly in				

B. Examine how well you are using your body mechanics when at work by completing the following form.

Recommended Technique	S	N.I.	U	Comments
Keep the work area as close to the body as possible				
Face the work area				
Keep the work area at a comfortable height				

(continued)

Recommended Technique	S	N.I.	U	Comments
Lower the body to reach a low work area; return to standing by lifting the body with the thigh and hip muscles				
Stand on a sturdy stool or stepladder when obtaining articles out of easy reach				
Pivot to turn the body				
Carry objects as close to the body as possible without contaminating the uniform				
Lean toward objects being pushed and away from objects being pulled				
Roll and slide objects rather than lift them whenever possible				
Use the longest and strongest muscles of the body				
Use an internal girdle and a long midriff				
Move muscles smoothly and evenly				
Maintain a good posture when working				
Rest after strenuous work or exercise				
Turning the Patient from His Back onto His Side				
Have the patient flex his knees and place his arms across his chest				
Place your hands on the patient's far shoulder and hip and gently roll the patient toward you				
Put up the bed siderails and move to the opposite side of the bed				
Move the patient's shoulders, then his hips, or both together if the patient is not heavy, to the center of the bed				
or				
Use techniques just described but roll the patient away from you, rather than toward you				
Turning the Patient toward You: Back onto His Abdomen				
Place the patient's arm near you under his buttock, palm up, and bring his far leg over the leg near you				
Turn the patient's face away from you				

Recommended Technique	S	N.I.	U	Comments
Grasp the patient's far hand and hip with your hands and gently roll the patient toward you onto his abdomen				
Move the patient into the center of the bed properly				
Turning the Patient Away from You: Back onto His Abdomen				
Put up the bed siderails on the far side of the bed and move the patient toward you				
Place the patient's arm away from you, under his buttock, palm up, and bring his near leg over his far leg				
Turn the patient's face toward you				
Place your arm under the patient's near leg and your other arm under the patient's far shoulder				
Gently roll the patient away from you onto his abdomen				
Turning the Patient from His Abdomen onto His Back				
Place the patient's far hand under his far thigh and cross his near leg over his far leg				
Turn the patient's face toward you				
Reach under the patient to grasp his far hand; place your other hand on his near hip				
Pull the patient's hand while pushing on his hip and gently roll him away from you onto his back				
or				
Place the patient's far hand under his far thigh and cross his near leg over his far leg				
Turn the patient's face toward you				
Put your arm between the patient's legs and thighs and place your hand on his far thigh				
Put your other arm under the patient's shoulders and place your hand on his far shoulder				
Straighten both of your arms as you gently roll the patient onto his back				

(continued)

Recommended Technique	S	N.I.	U	Comments
Moving the Patient Up in Bed				
Remove pillows from under the patient's head and place one against the bed's headboard				
Have the patient flex his knees; place one of your arms under the patient's shoulders and the other under his hip				
Using a wide base of support, rock toward the head of the bed as the patient pushes with his feet				
Obtain an assistant if the patient is too heavy for one person to move				
The Three-Carrier Lift				
Place the stretcher at a right angle to the foot of the bed and lock its wheels				
Place the tallest carrier at the patient's head and shoulders, the other two at his legs and waist				
Have the three carriers place their hands well under the patient and have them move him to the near side of the bed				
Have the three carriers logroll the patient onto their chests and then pivot toward the stretcher				
Carry the patient to the stretcher and gently place him on it				

C. This section allows you to examine your techniques for assisting the patient with positioning.

Recommended Technique	S	N.I.	U	Comments
The Back-Lying Position				
Place a small pillow under the patient's upper shoulders, neck, and head; cervical spine is extended				
Bring the arms out to the side, flex the elbows, and place the forearms on pillows in pronation				
Extend the wrists and place a handroll in the patient's hands, as indicated				
See to it that the wrists are above the level of the elbows and the elbows are above shoulder level				
Place a small roll at the proximal area under the knees so that they are only slightly flexed				
Use a footboard to support the patient's feet at right angles to his lower legs				

Recommended Technique	S	N.I.	U	Comments
Place sandbags or trochanter rolls alongside the patient's hips and thighs				
Arrange top bed linens over the footboard in a way so they do not rest on the feet				
The Side-Lying Position				
Place a small pillow under the patient's neck so that the neck is in a position of extension				
Place the patient's arm on the side on which he is lying so that the elbow is flexed about 90°				
Place the flexed arm alongside a pillow at the patient's head				
Place a pillow under the arm on the opposite side on which the patient is lying				
Slightly flex the knee on the side on which the patient is lying				
Place pillow(s) under the thigh, leg, and foot of the leg opposite the side on which the patient is lying, and flex the knee slightly				
Pull the hip on which the patient is lying backward slightly				
The Face-Lying Position				
Move the patient down in bed after he is on his abdomen so that his feet are over the edge of the mattress				
or				
Instead of the above technique, support the legs on pillows so that the toes do not touch the bed				
Place the patient's arms alongside his head or body, depending on the patient's comfort				
Place a very small pillow under the patient's head if the patient finds this comfortable				
Slip a small pillow under the patient between the bottom ribs and the upper abdomen if the patient finds this comfortable				

(continued)

Recommended Technique	S	N.I.	U	Comments
Fowler's Position				
Raise the head of the bed to the desired height				
Allow the patient's head to rest against the mattress or on a small pillow, depending on comfort				
Position the patient so that the angle of elevation begins at the hips				
Support the forearms on pillows so that they are elevated enough to prevent a pull on the patient's shoulders				
Support the hands on pillows so that they are in natural alignment with the forearms higher than the elbows				
Elevate the knees a bit for short periods of time only, if this adds to the patient's comfort				
Support the feet at right angles to the lower legs and keep top bed linens off the patient's toes				

PERFORMANCE CHECKLIST

A. This section allows you to examine your techniques for assisting with range-of-motion exercises.
1. Place a check mark in the "S" ("satisfactory") column if you used the recommended technique.
2. Place a check mark in the "N.I." ("needs improvement") column if you used some but not all of each recommended technique.
3. Place a check mark in the "U" ("unsatisfactory") column if you forgot to include that particular recommended technique.
4. The section for comment allows space to make notes about when further practice is indicated, what errors you made, suggestions that will improve your skills, and so on.

Recommended Technique	S	N.I.	U	Comments
Know the patient's diagnosis and why the exercises are used				
Explain to the patient what exercise will be used, why it is used, and how it will be done				
Avoid overexertion and do not fatigue the patient				
Start exercising gradually and work slowly with smooth, rhythmic, and regular motions				
Use a firm but comfortable grip on the patient when moving body parts				
Move the joint until there is resistance but no pain				
Support the part being exercised well at the proximal parts of the joints, do not grasp muscle groups				
Return the joint to a neutral position when finishing each exercise				
Stop the exercises if spasticity of muscles occurs				
Keep friction at a minimum when moving the extremities				
Use the exercises as prescribed, usually two times a day				
Do each exercise two to five times, depending on the patient's needs				
Check the patient's respiratory and pulse rates and evaluate when the exercising may be too strenuous				

(continued)

Recommended Technique	S	N.I.	U	Comments
Use passive exercises as necessary but encourage the patient to use active exercises when possible				
Extend, hyperextend, flex, and rotate the neck, back, shoulder, and hip joints appropriately				
Abduct and adduct the arms				
Extend, hyperextend, flex, and rotate the elbow, wrist, finger, and thumb joints appropriately				
Abduct and adduct the legs				
Extend, hyperextend, flex, and rotate the knee, ankle, and toe joints appropriately				
Observe any special orders when conducting range-of-motion exercises				

B. This section allows you to examine your techniques for using a continuous passive motion machine.

Recommended Technique	S	N.I.	U	Comments
Review the exercise prescription for the patient				
Determine the patient's need for pain-relieving medication before you start				
Develop a schedule with the patient for using the machine				
Obtain the CPM machine and a piece of sheepskin for making a cradle for the calf				
Wear gloves to empty any wound-drainage containers and change dressing				
Wash your hands				
Explain the procedure to the patient				
Position the patient appropriately for comfort during the exercise period				
Place the machine on the bed and position the patient appropriately				
Position the knee correctly				
Support and stabilize the leg				
Adjust machine to a lower prescribed rate and turn it on				
Observe the patient's response				

Recommended Technique	S	N.I.	U	Comments
Readjust the alignment of the leg or the position of the machine as needed				
Increase the degree of flexion and number of cycles gradually to prescribed levels				
Turn machine off at end of exercise period with leg extended				
Release straps; support joints at knee and ankle while lifting leg				
Remove machine; Encourage active range-of-motion and isometric exercises				
Document assessment data, use of machine, level of exercise, and patient's response				

CHAPTER 25

Mechanical Immobilization

SUMMARY

Mechanical immobilization is used for patients who have sustained trauma to the musculoskeletal system. These injuries are painful and do not heal as rapidly as the skin or soft tissue does. They require a period of inactivity during the time that the body requires to repair the damaged structures.

Treatment requires mechanical immobilization devices that cover, attach to, and confine areas of the body for varying and extended periods of time. The purpose of these devices is to inactivate the injured area and prevent further trauma while avoiding injury to other body structures while they are used. This chapter describes the specialized skills and techniques needed to care for patients who require mechanical immobilization.

MATCHING QUESTIONS

Directions: For items 1 through 6 match the descriptions in Part B with the devices in Part A.

Part A

1. _____ Braces
2. _____ Cast
3. _____ Immobilizer
4. _____ Sling
5. _____ Splint
6. _____ Petal

Part B

a. Device that immobilizes an injured body part
b. Cloth device used to elevate, cradle, and support
c. Custom-made devices designed to support weak structures
d. Adhesive tape reinforcement to protect the skin
e. A rigid mold placed around a body part
f. Commercial splint made from cloth or foam

MULTIPLE CHOICE QUESTIONS

Directions: For items 1 through 10, circle the letter that corresponds to the best answer for each question.

1. A device that is used to support or align a body part and prevent or correct deformities is called a(an):
   a. Windows
   b. Functional brace
   c. External fixator
   d. Orthoses

2. A foam or rigid splint used to treat athletic neck injuries is called a(an):
   a. Molder splint
   b. Internal fixator
   c. Cervical collar
   d. Brace

3. When applying a splinting device to an injured lower leg, the device should extend:
   a. From mid-thigh to the ankle
   b. From below the knee to the ankle
   c. From mid-thigh to below the ankle
   d. From below the knee to the toes

4. Which of the following is the first action when applying a triangular sling to support an injured arm:
   a. Place the upper end of the base of the triangle around the back of the neck on the unaffected side
   b. Place the upper end of the base of the triangle around the back of the neck on the affected side
   c. Place the open triangle on the patient's chest with the base of the triangle along the length of the patient's chest on the unaffected side
   d. Place the open triangle on the patient's chest with the base of the triangle along the length of the patient's chest on the affected side

5. Newly applied plaster casts may remain wet for:
   a. 24 to 48 hours
   b. 24 to 36 hours
   c. 20 to 30 hours
   d. 12 to 24 hours

6. The most appropriate way to dry a plaster cast is to:
   a. Expose the surface to a heat cradle
   b. Use an electric fan to circulate air on it
   c. Apply electric heating pads to the surface
   d. Expose the surface to room air circulation

7. Following surgery and the application of a cast, the nurse's primary concern should be:
   a. Assessing for pain and discomfort
   b. Assessing for swelling and bleeding
   c. Assessing the cast for hot spots
   d. Assessing the cast for wetness

8. An assessment technique recommended for determining the extent and effects of swelling and circulation of a casted area is:
   a. Assessing the pulse
   b. Assessing the blood pressure
   c. Assessing capillary refill
   d. Assessing level of pain

9. To avoid compromised circulation to an area protected by a pneumatic splint, examination and treatment should take place within:
   a. 5–15 minutes
   b. 15–30 minutes
   c. 30–45 minutes
   d. 45–60 minutes

10. Custom-made devices that are designed to support weakened structures during periods of activity are called:
    a. Braces
    b. Splints
    c. Slings
    d. Casts

TRUE OR FALSE QUESTIONS

Directions: For items 1 through 12, decide if the statement is true or false and mark T or F in the space provided.

1. _____ A splint is a device designed to support weakened body structures during weight bearing.

2. _____ Pneumatic and traction splints are intended for brief periods of use immediately after an injury.

3. _____ A pneumatic splint should be fully inflated to produce sufficient pressure on the injured area.

4. _____ Casts made of the newer synthetic materials take 24 to 48 hours to dry.

5. _____ The nurse should use only the palms of the hands to move and reposition the cast while it is wet.

6. _____ A wet cast should be covered to protect the patient from chilling.

7. _____ The blanching test is used to assess the warmth of tissues.

8. _____ Bleeding under a cast is characterized by dark red areas on the cast.

9. _____ Rough edges of a cast may be repaired by applying petals made from adhesive tape.

10. _____ The electric cast saw must be used by a physician because it will cut the patient's skin.

11. _____ Following cast removal, the skin should be scrubbed to forcibly remove the loose skin.

12. _____ Patients in skeletal traction must avoid active range of motion.

SHORT ANSWER QUESTIONS

Directions: Read each of the following statements and supply the word(s) necessary in the space provided.

1. Identify the five general purposes of mechanical immobilization.
   a. _____
   b. _____
   c. _____
   d. _____
   e. _____

2. Identify ten of the important techniques that should be followed when applying an emergency splint.
   a. _____
   b _____
   c. _____
   d. _____
   e. _____
   f. _____
   g. _____
   h. _____
   i. _____
   j. _____

3. List the three types of casts.

   a. _____

   b. _____

   c. _____

4. Identify four principles for maintaining effective traction.

   a. _____

   b. _____

   c. _____

   d. _____

CRITICAL THINKING EXERCISE

Prepare a teaching plan for a patient who is right-handed with a broken right wrist that has been casted. Complete the following form.

Topic for Teaching	Points to Cover in a Teaching Program
Accommodations necessary for:	
a. eating	
b. dressing	
c. hygiene	
d. toileting	
e. working	

PERFORMANCE CHECKLIST

A. This section allows you to examine your techniques for caring for the patient who has a cast.
1. Place a check mark in the "S" ("satisfactory") column if you used the recommended technique.
2. Place a check mark in the "N.I." ("needs improvement") column if you used some but not all of each recommended technique.

3. Place a check mark in the "U" ("unsatisfactory") column if you forgot to include that particular recommended technique.
4. The section for comment allows space to make notes about when further practice is indicated, what errors you made, suggestions that will improve your skills, and so on.

Recommended Technique	S	N.I.	U	Comments
Know the type of fracture the patient has and why a particular type of cast was applied				
Elevate the cast and allow nothing to rest on it				
Expose the cast to air or use appropriate devices to promote drying of a new fiberglass cast				
Look for signs/symptoms that indicate the cast is too tight				
Look for signs/symptoms that indicate there is bleeding under the cast				
Look for signs/symptoms that indicate there is an infection in tissues under the cast				
Make the above three observations at frequent intervals, the first two at least every hour during the first 24 hours				
Report any unusual signs or symptoms promptly				
Petal a cast properly				
Keep the cast clean and do not introduce various devices under the cast				
Protect a cast placed near the perineal area appropriately				
Use range-of-motion and isometric exercises				
Teach the patient and family about proper cast care				

(continued)

B. This section allows you to examine your technique while caring for the patient in traction

Recommended Technique	S	N.I.	U	Comments
Inspect the mechanical equipment for the application of traction				
Provide a trapeze if the type of traction allows the patient to raise her body weight				
Position or reposition the patient so that her body is centered in the bed and the body part in traction is in the same line of pull				
Avoid tucking top linens beneath the mattress				
Instruct the patient and nursing personnel as to the length of time the patient is to be attached to the traction				
Identify the positions that the patient may assume				
Wash and rub posterior parts of the body by depressing the mattress				
Make the bed by removing bottom linens from head toward toes				
Provide pressure-relieving devices under bony prominences				
Apply elbow and heel protectors as needed				
Omit the use of pillows unless specified				
Provide fracture bedpan for bowel elimination if lifting the hips alters the line of pull				
Encourage active range of motion and isometric and isotonic exercises as much as possible				
Encourage frequent dorsiflexion of unrestricted lower extremities				
Inspect the skin for potential and possible areas of irritation and breakdown frequently				
Cleanse the skin around skeletal pin-insertion sites and apply antimicrobial agents as ordered				
Apply or change dressings around skeletal pin-insertion sites using sterile technique				
Cover any sharp points on traction devices				
Assess the color, temperature, and mobility of all areas where traction is applied				
Record the frequency of bowel movements				
Provide diversional activities as necessary				

CHAPTER 26

Ambulatory Aids

SUMMARY

This chapter provides information on the nursing activities and mechanical devices used to promote mobility in debilitated patients. Activities to prepare the patient for ambulation and exercises to strengthen and tone muscles are described.

MATCHING QUESTIONS

Directions: For items 1 through 4, match the methods of use in Part B with the crutch-walking gaits in Part A.

Part A
1. _____ Two-point gait
2. _____ Three-point gait
3. _____ Four-point gait
4. _____ Swing-through

Part B
a. Only one point is moved forward at a time (i.e., left crutch, right foot, right crutch, left foot, etc.).
b. The crutches are advanced together. The body weight is shifted from the legs to the hand grips. The legs are swung either slightly beyond or parallel with the crutches.
c. The patient bears weight on both feet. The right crutch and the left foot are moved forward. Then, the left foot and right crutch move forward.
d. Both crutches and the leg that cannot bear weight move forward and then the foot permitted to bear weight comes through.

MULTIPLE CHOICE QUESTIONS

Directions: For items 1 through 10, circle the letter that corresponds to the best answer for each question.

1. Muscle tone refers to:
   a. The muscle's ability to respond
   b. The muscle's power to perform
   c. The muscle's ability to contract
   d. The muscle's strength at rest

2. Quadriceps setting is an example of:
   a. Isotonic exercise
   b. Aerobic exercise
   c. Isometric exercise
   d. Passive exercise

3. For optimum use, a cane must be adjusted to an appropriate height for the patient as follows:
   a. The handle should be parallel with the patient's hip allowing the elbow to extend
   b. The handle should be parallel with the patient's hip allowing 15 degrees of elbow flexion
   c. The handle should allow the patient to lean forward 15 degrees with the elbow flexed 10 degrees
   d. The handle should allow the patient to stand straight with the elbow flexed 15 degrees

4. Patients who require the use of crutches for ambulation but who are unable to bear weight on their hands and wrists would most likely use:
   a. Lofstrand crutches
   b. Axillary crutches
   c. Canadian crutches
   d. Platform crutches

5. The most stable form of ambulatory aid is:
   a. A cane
   b. Crutches
   c. A walking belt
   d. A walker

6. Quadriceps setting is done in which of the following ways:
   a. The patient pinches the buttocks together and then relaxes
   b. The patient sits in bed and raises his buttocks up by pushing down with his hands
   c. The patient lies on his abdomen and lifts his head and shoulders off the bed with his arms
   d. The patient pulls the kneecaps toward the hips by pushing down on his knees

7. When a patient is using a cane, he should:
   a. Place the cane about 10 centimeters (4 inches) to the side of the foot and hold it on the involved side
   b. Place the cane about 10 centimeters (4 inches) to the side of the foot and hold it on the uninvolved side
   c. Place the cane about 5 centimeters (2.5 inches) to the side of the foot and hold it on the involved side.
   d. Place the cane about 5 centimeters (2.5 inches) to the side of the foot and hold it on the uninvolved side.

8. In which of the following situations would the individual use the three-point gait for crutch walking:
   a. The patient must be able to bear some weight on each leg
   b. Weight bearing is allowed on one leg and no weight or only limited weight on the other leg
   c. Weight bearing must be permitted on both feet, but they may have weak or limited ability
   d. One or both legs are involved and the patient usually has leg braces or a cast

9. Which of the following are appropriate for walking on stairs with a cane:
   a. Use the cane rather than the stair rail
   b. Keep your back straight
   c. Going up take each step with the stronger leg first
   d. Move cane forward with the stronger extremity

10. When using a walker, patients are instructed to:
   a. Stand within the walker
   b. Advance the walker 10 to 12 inches
   c. Always step with the stronger extremity
   d. Flex their hips and knees when walking

TRUE OR FALSE QUESTIONS

Directions: For items 1 through 10, decide if the statement is true or false and mark T or F in the space provided.

1. _____ Most patients are capable of performing quadriceps and gluteal setting exercises independently.

2. _____ The nurse should place a rolled towel under the knees before the patient attempts the quadriceps setting exercise.

3. _____ Crutches should fit snugly into the patient's axilla to prevent her from falling.

4. _____ A cane is a hand-held device that is used by patients who have weakness on one side of their body.

5. _____ When assisting a patient to ambulate using a walking belt, the nurse should hold on to the handles of the belt and walk behind the patient.

6. _____ It is possible to obtain an approximate measurement for crutch length by subtracting 40 centimeters from the patient's height.

7. _____ In older adults, postural changes may result in a swaying or shuffling gait.

8. _____ When walking down stairs while using a cane, take each step with the stronger leg first.

9. _____ A walker is the most stable form of ambulatory aid.

10. _____ Antiembolism stockings are not necessary for patients being placed on a tilt table for pre-ambulation therapy.

SHORT ANSWER QUESTIONS

Directions: Read each of the following statements and supply the word(s) necessary in the space provided.

1. List four devices and techniques that provide support and assistance with walking.
   a. _____
   b. _____
   c. _____
   d. _____

2. List three common aids for ambulation.
   a. _____
   b. _____
   c. _____

3. Describe three characteristics of appropriately fitted crutches.
   a. _____
   b. _____
   c. _____

4. Explain the reason for using a tilt table as part of perambulation therapy.

CRITICAL THINKING EXERCISE

Describe how the nurse could demonstrate respect for individual decision making when the patients requiring the use of ambulatory aids are of pre-school age, an adolescent, and an older adult.

   a. Pre-school age

   b. Adolescent

   c. Older adult

PERFORMANCE CHECKLIST

A. This section allows you to examine your techniques for caring for the patient who has an ambulatory aid or needs assistance with ambulation.

1. Place a check mark in the "S" ("satisfactory") column if you used the recommended technique.
2. Place a check mark in the "N.I." ("needs improvement") column if you used some but not all of each recommended technique.

3. Place a check mark in the "U" ("unsatisfactory") column if you forgot to include that particular recommended technique.
4. The section for comment allows space to make notes about when further practice is indicated, what errors you made, suggestions that will improve your skills, and so on.

Recommended Technique	S	N.I.	U	Comments
Have the patient use quadriceps drills by having him contract and relax muscles on the front of the thigh				
Have the patient fix his buttocks by pinching them together and then relaxing them				
Use push-ups properly as indicated if this exercise is recommended				
Prepare the patient for dangling by placing him in Fowler's position for a few minutes				
Pivot the patient so that his legs dangle over the edge of the bed, feet resting on a footstool or on the floor				
Assist the patient to a chair properly. Walk alongside the patient using a walking belt when he is ready to ambulate				
Demonstrate the proper use of a walking belt, a cane, and crutches when the patient requires these devices				

B. This section allows you to examine your techniques for assisting with crutch walking.

Recommended Technique	S	N.I.	U	Comments
Review the medical orders for the type of activity and crutch-walking gait				
Observe the condition of the patient's axilla and palms				

(continued)

Recommended Technique	S	N.I.	U	Comments
Inspect the condition of the axillary pads and rubber crutch tips				
Ask if there are any symptoms such as pain, numbness, or tingling in the fingers or joints				
Assist the patient to put on a robe, clothing, and appropriate walking shoes				
Apply a walking belt as necessary				
Clear the pathway where the patient will walk				
Wash your hands				
Assist the patient to a standing position				
Offer the crutches and observe that they are placed correctly				
Remind the patient to stand straight with the shoulders relaxed				
Position yourself to the side and slightly behind the patient				
Position yourself on the patient's weaker side				
Instruct the patient to move forward				
Observe that the patient uses the prescribed gait				
Stop if there is evidence of fatigue or intolerance for the activity				
Evaluate the patient's tolerance of the activity				
Document the activity				

CHAPTER 27

Perioperative Care

SUMMARY

Certain illnesses must be treated through surgery. Surgery involves the entering of tissues and removal or reconstructing of structures that are diseased, injured, or malformed. This chapter discusses basic care of the surgical patient. It includes care that applies, in general, to all surgical patients, regardless of diagnosis or type of surgery. The discussion also includes laser surgery and blood donors from autologous and directed donor sources.

MATCHING QUESTIONS

Directions: For items 1 through 5, match the examples in Part B with the types of surgery in Part A.

Part A
1. _____ Optional
2. _____ Elective
3. _____ Required
4. _____ Urgent
5. _____ Emergency

Part B
a. Surgery for the removal of a cataract
b. Surgery to relieve an intestinal obstruction
c. Surgery for the removal of a superficial cyst
d. Surgery for cosmetic purposes
e. Surgery for the removal of a malignant tumor

Directions: For items 6 through 12, match the descriptions in Part B with the complications in Part A.

Part A
6. _____ Airway occlusion
7. _____ Evisceration
8. _____ Adynamic ileus
9. _____ Hypoxemia
10. _____ Urinary retention
11. _____ Dehiscence
12. _____ Shock

Part B
a. Inadequate oxygenation of blood
b. Severe rapid blood loss
c. Obstruction of trachea from swelling
d. Inability to void
e. Separation of incision
f. Lack of bowel motility
g. Protrusion of abdominal organs through incision
h. Inadequate blood flow

MULTIPLE CHOICE QUESTIONS

Directions: For items 1 through 10, circle the letter that corresponds to the best answer for each question.

1. Which of the following is the primary disadvantage of outpatient surgery:
   a. It requires that care of the patient following discharge be carried out by unskilled individuals
   b. It allows for fewer delays in assessing and preparing a patient once she arrives for surgery
   c. It requires intensive preoperative teaching in a short amount of time
   d. It reduces the time for establishing a nurse-patient relationship

2. With which type of anesthesia does the patient experience loss of feeling in the lower half of the body only:
   a. General anesthesia
   b. Regional anesthesia
   c. Local anesthesia
   d. Topical anesthesia

3. Which of the following is true of directed donors:
   a. They must be at least 21 years old
   b. They must meet volunteer donor medical history criteria
   c. They must weigh at least 95 pounds
   d. They may donate one unit every 56 days

4. A postoperative patient's question, "How am I doing?" may really mean:
   a. "I'm doing fine, don't you think?"
   b. "I'm worried about my family."
   c. "Is the surgery all over?"
   d. "Do you think I'll make it?"

5. The postoperative complication that deep-breathing exercises help most to prevent is:
   a. Hiccups
   b. Phlebitis
   c. Atelectasis
   d. Nausea

6. Which type of cough should the patient be taught to use postoperatively:
   a. Hard
   b. Hacking
   c. Whooping
   d. Forced

7. To prevent the formation of thrombi and emboli in the postoperative patient, the nurse should:
   a. Have the patient lie still
   b. Place pillows under the knees
   c. Raise the knee gatch
   d. Teach foot and leg exercises

8. Mr. J states that he is worried about his planned operation. Of the following comments the nurse can make, which would be the most appropriate response?
   a. "Don't worry, Mr. J. Your surgeon has done this many times."
   b. "There is really no need to worry; it will be Ok."
   c. "Tell me what worries you about the surgery."
   d. "Mrs. S. had the same surgery yesterday and she is fine"

9. Plume produced during laser surgery can be hazardous because the:
   a. Smell is damaging to the nasal tissues
   b. Smoke may cause burning and watering of the eyes
   c. Airborne cells and viruses may be inhaled
   d. Water may produce routes for contamination

10. When a 7-year-old male patient states that he doesn't want to cry after his operation, the nurse's best response would be:
    a. "It is all right if you cry."
    b. "Big boys don't cry."
    c. "It will not help if you cry."
    d. "Crying will only make things worse."

TRUE OR FALSE QUESTIONS

Directions: For items 1 through 15, decide if the statement is true or false and mark T or F in the space provided.

1. _____ The separation of a wound with exposure of body organs is known as dehiscence.

2. _____ Patients scheduled for outpatient surgery must check into the hospital the night before.

3. _____ The nurse shares the responsibility for assessing factors that pose a hazard for the patient undergoing surgery.

4. _____ An autologous transfusion is made from one's own blood.

5. _____ Shaving the surgical area the night before surgery is the safest method for preventing the growth of microorganisms.

6. _____ The individual who is donating blood as a directed donor must weight at least 95 pounds.

7. _____ An individual designated as a directed donor may give blood once every week.

8. _____ It is generally agreed that forced coughing should be routinely performed postoperatively.

9. _____ It is a nursing responsibility to check that a surgical consent has been obtained before proceeding with the preparation of a patient for surgery.

10. _____ The special skin preparation prior to surgery is done to sterilize the skin.

11. _____ The nurse who is caring for the preoperative patient is responsible for checking to make sure all the items on the preoperative checklist have been completed.

12. _____ It is important to give the operative patient's family the exact time their family member will return from the recovery room.

13. _____ When teaching patients deep-breathing, the nurse should emphasize that the breathing should be done rapidly.

14. _____ It is best to apply antiembolism stockings after the patient has been out of bed and has exercised his legs.
15. _____ Hypovolemic shock is caused by blood loss due to hemorrhage.

SHORT ANSWER QUESTIONS

Directions: Read each of the following statements and supply the word(s) necessary in the space provided.

1. List the equipment and supplies that are likely to be needed in readiness for the postoperative patient's room as suggested in this chapter.
   a. _____
   b. _____
   c. _____
   d. _____

2. List the advantages of laser surgery suggested in this chapter.
   a. _____
   b. _____
   c. _____
   d. _____
   e. _____
   f. _____
   g. _____
   h. _____
   i. _____

3. List six areas commonly addressed in discharge instructions.
   a. _____
   b. _____
   c. _____
   d. _____
   e. _____
   f. _____

4. Identify eight general types of measures included in postoperative orders as suggested in this chapter.
   a. _____
   b. _____
   c. _____
   d. _____
   e. _____
   f. _____
   g. _____
   h. _____

CRITICAL THINKING EXERCISES

1. Describe adjustments you make when caring for preoperative and postoperative patients:
   a. When the patient is an infant or child

   b. When the patient has diabetes mellitus

   c. When the patient is obese

   d. When the patient is elderly

PERFORMANCE CHECKLIST

A. This section allows you to examine your techniques for caring for the patient who has surgery.

1. Place a check mark in the "S" ("satisfactory") column if you used the recommended technique.
2. Place a check mark in the "N.I." ("needs improvement") column if you used some but not all of each recommended technique.
3. Place a check mark in the "U" ("unsatisfactory") column if you forgot to include that particular recommended technique.
4. The section for comment allows space to make notes about when further practice is indicated, what errors you made, suggestions that will improve your skills, and so on.

Recommended Technique	S	N.I.	U	Comments
Changing position of the patient				
Increasing activity for the patient				
Preparing the patient for ambulation				
Helping the patient to walk				
Having the patient perform self-care				
Other topics, depending on patients needs				
Teaching Deep-Breathing				
Position the patient for comfort				
Help the patient relax to allow for total lung expansion				
Have the patient take a deep breath to the count of five to seven, with 1 second per count				
Teach the patient to make her abdomen larger while inhaling				
Have the patient hold her breath to the count of three after inhaling deeply				
Have the patient exhale against pursed lips for about twice as long as it took her to inhale				
Teach the patient to contract her abdomen toward her spine while exhaling				
Repeat inhaling and exhaling several times with a few seconds rest between respirations				

(continued)

Recommended Technique	S	N.I.	U	Comments
Watch for signs that the patient may be breathing too rapidly and instruct her to rest between breaths				
Have the patient practice deep-breathing until she is able to do so correctly				
Teach the patient how to use incentive spirometry with equipment of the agency's choice				
Teaching Leg and Foot Exercises				
Have the patient positioned on her back				
Teach the patient to bend one knee, raise the foot, hold the position, and then extend the leg				
Have the patient do the same exercise with the other leg				
Have the patient draw imaginary circles with the great toes				
Have the patient repeat the exercise five times every two hours				
Teaching Coughing				
Determine what the patient will be able to do postoperatively in relation to coughing				
Position the patient in Fowler's position, unless contraindicated				
Splint the area well where the operative site will be				
Have the patient inhale deeply and then have her give two or three forced coughs				
Have the patient cough three times in a row while exhaling				
Follow the coughing with a deep breath and cough again if secretions remain				
Miscellaneous Preoperative Teaching				
The use of a bedpan and urinal				
Commonly used tubes				
Frequency of vital signs				
Measures to control discomfort and sleeplessness				

Recommended Technique	S	N.I.	U	Comments
Diet and fluid restrictions				
Immediate preoperative and postoperative care				
Visiting privileges				

B. This section allows you to examine your techniques for preparing a patient for a surgical procedure

Recommended Technique	S	N.I	U	Comments
Note that the patient has had a complete examination and is familiar with his condition				
Assist with measures to help the patient so that he is well rested and in a good nutritional state				
Note that the proper consent for surgery has been completed				
Check vital signs preoperatively, including immediately before surgery, and report abnormalities promptly				
See to it that the incisional area is properly prepared, including shaving the area as necessary				
Administer a cleansing enema preoperatively if ordered				
Attend to the patient's hygienic needs the night before and immediately before surgery				
Administer prescribed medications the day/night before and immediately before surgery				
See to it that the patient has had nothing by mouth as ordered				
Care for the patient's valuables according to agency policy				
Remove the patient's cosmetics, hairpins, and hair clips; secure long hair in place				
Gown and cap the patient for surgery; use stockings if agency policy requires				
See to it that the patient voids immediately before surgery and report promptly if he does not				
Assist with transferring the patient to surgery and check the patient's identity with operating-room personnel				

(continued)

C. This section allows you to examine your techniques for receiving a patient from the recovery room.

Recommended Technique	S	N.I.	U	Comments
Have the room and bed ready to receive the patient				
Verify the identity of the patient with recovery-room personnel				
Assist recovery-room personnel to transfer the patient to his bed				
Position the patient properly in bed				
Obtain a report on the patient's condition from recovery-room personnel				
Check the patient's vital signs, including skin color, and report anything unusual				
Check the dressings for evidence of excessive bleeding and report unusual findings				
Check the patient's postoperative orders and carry out those that need to be taken care of immediately				
Check the patient for level of consciousness and help him to become oriented				
Put bed siderails in place and leave the signal device handy when it is safe to leave the patient				
Notify relatives that the patient has returned from surgery and tell them when they may visit with him				
Continue to check the patient's vital signs, level of consciousness, and dressings according to agency policy				

D. This section allows you to examine your techniques for applying antiembolism stockings.

Recommended Technique	S	N.I.	U	Comments
Use the manufacturer's instructions to see to it that the patient has properly fitting stockings				
Plan to apply the stockings before the patient is out of bed in the morning				
Check to see that the patient's legs are dry and clean before applying the stockings				
Use powder or cornstarch on the skin, as indicated; avoid massaging the legs				

Recommended Technique	S	N.I.	U	Comments
Put on the stockings according to the manufacturer's instructions				
Check to see that heels are properly placed in the stockings and that toes are not under pressure				
Avoid turning down the top of the stockings and see to it that they are free of wrinkles				
Check the legs regularly, two or three times a day, for redness, blistering, swelling, pain, and so on				
Remove the stockings at least once a shift to check and bathe the legs and feet				
See to it that the stockings are laundered as necessary				

PERFORMANCE CHECKLIST

A. This section allows you to examine your techniques for caring for the patient who requires a dressing change.
  1. Place a check mark in the "S" ("satisfactory") column if you used the recommended technique.
  2. Place a check mark in the "N.I. " ("needs improvement") column if you used some but not all of each recommended technique.

3. Place a check mark in the "U" ("unsatisfactory") column if you forgot to include that particular recommended technique.
4. The section for comment allows space to make notes about when further practice is indicated, what errors you made, suggestions that will improve your skills, and so on.

Recommended Technique	S.	N.I.	U	Comments
Set up a sterile field with all necessary supplies and equipment				
Remove adhesive securing the dressing while pulling it toward the wound				
Remove and discard the soiled dressings in a waterproof container				
If the dressing sticks to the wound, moisten it with sterile water or normal saline				
Cleanse the wound with the antiseptic of the agency's choice				
Allow the antiseptic to dry before applying fresh dressings				
Inspect the wound carefully and note any abnormalities				
Cover the wound with sterile dressings				
Secure the dressing in place appropriately				
Use gloves according to agency policy; observe aseptic technique throughout the procedure				

B. This section allows you to examine your techniques for irrigating a wound, shortening a drain, packing a wound, and dressing a draining wound.

Recommended Technique	S.	N.I.	U	Comments
Assemble necessary sterile equipment, including sterile solution for the irrigation				
Position and drape the patient appropriately				

(continued)

Recommended Technique	S.	N.I.	U	Comments
Remove adhesive securing the dressing while pulling it toward the wound				
Remove and discard the soiled dressings in a waterproof container				
Prepare the prescribed solution for the wound irrigation correctly				
Remove and discard the soiled dressing appropriately				
Inspect the wound carefully and estimate amount of drainage				
Position the patient so that solution will flow from the wound into a collecting basin				
Irrigate the wound generously but carefully, being sure to irrigate pockets in the wound				
If a drain is present, shorten it correctly as prescribed				
If the wound needs packing, pack it well as prescribed				
Clean the wound and the skin immediately around it with cotton balls and the antiseptic of the agency's choice				
Move the cotton balls away from the wound's center, or toward it if heavily contaminated, following agency policy				
Allow the wound to dry and apply skin protectant of the agency's choice, as indicated				
Apply a wet-to-dry dressing appropriately and as prescribed				
If wet-to-dry dressings are not used, cover the wound with sterile dressings				
Fluff and loosely pack dressing, depending on the amount of drainage				
Secure the dressing				
Use gloves according to agency policy; observe aseptic technique throughout the procedure				
See that the dressing is changed often enough to prevent it from becoming soaked				

C. This section allows you to examine your techniques for using various bandages and binders.

Recommended Technique	S.	N.I.	U	Comments
Use porous rather than nonporous materials when possible to allow air circulation at the area of application				
Use powder to decrease friction, but only on unbroken skin and well away from a wound				
Do not allow skin surfaces to touch each other under bandages and binders				
Pad bony prominences under bandages and binders				
Place the part to be bandaged comfortably and in its normal anatomic position				
Apply bandages and binders securely but not so tightly that they interfere with circulation or breathing				
Use bandages and binders on extremities in a way so that toes and fingers are exposed				
Apply bandages and binders so that considerable portions of extremities are not exposed				
Bandage an extremity toward the trunk of the body				
Be careful not to apply a bandage or binder too tightly over a draining area				
Avoid excessively thick or extensive bandages and binders				
Check bandages and binders regularly to see to it that there is no interference with circulation or breathing				
Demonstrate ability to use various turns correctly when applying roller bandages:				
Circular turn				
Spiral turn				
Spiral-reverse turn				
Figure-of-eight turn				
Spica				
Recurrent turn				

(continued)

Recommended Technique	S.	N.I.	U	Comments
Demonstrate ability to use various types of binders correctly:				
T binder tailed binder				
Scultetus binder				
Straight binder				
Triangular binder				
Cravat binder				

CHAPTER 29

Gastrointestinal Intubation

SUMMARY

Intubation is the term used for placing a tube into a structure of the body. When the tube is inserted into the stomach by passing it through the nose or mouth, it is called gastric intubation. If the tube passes through the intestinal tract and stops after it exits the stomach, it is called intestinal intubation. Tubes may also be inserted through a surgically created opening called an ostomy. Certain patients, especially those experiencing abdominal or gastrointestinal surgery, may require the placement of such a tube. This chapter discusses the uses for gastrointestinal tubes and the nursing guidelines and skills required for managing patient care in these situations.

MATCHING QUESTIONS

Directions: For items 1 through 6, match the purposes in Part B with the types of gastrointestinal tubes in Part A.

Part A
1. _____   Ewald
2. _____   Levin
3. _____   Salem sump
4. _____   Sengstaken-Blakemore
5. _____   Keofeed
6. _____   Cantor

Part B
a. Intestinal decompression
b. Decompression
c. Lavage
d. Compression
e. Diagnostics
f. Gavage

Directions: For items 7 through 10, match the disadvantages in Part B with the feeding tubes in Part A.

Part A
7. _____   Nasogastric
8. _____   Nasointestinal
9. _____   Gastrostomy
10. _____   Jejunostomy

Part B
a. Must wait 24 hours after initial placement to use
b. Potentiates gastric reflux
c. Increased incidence for infection
d. Requires x-ray to verify placement

Directions: For items 11 through 20, match the solutions in Part B with the problem in part A.

Part A
11. _____   Diarrhea
12. _____   Nausea and vomiting
13. _____   Aspiration
14. _____   Constipation
15. _____   Elevated blood glucose
16. _____   Middle ear inflammation
17. _____   Sore throat
18. _____   Plugged feeding tube
19. _____   Dumping syndrome
20. _____   Elevated electrolytes

Part B
a. Check placement before instilling liquids
b. Administer small, continuous volume
c. Increase supplemental water
d. Hang only 4 hours' worth of formula
e. Dilute crushed drugs
f. Change formula
g. Change position every 2 hours
h. Increase concentration
i. Allow feeding to instill by gravity
j. Use smaller tube

183

MULTIPLE CHOICE QUESTIONS
•••••••••••••••••••••••••••••••••••••••

Directions: For items 1 through 15, circle the letter that corresponds to the best answer for each question.

1. Highly concentrated tube feedings can result in:
    a. Constipation
    b. Nausea and vomiting
    c. Aspiration
    d. Diarrhea

2. Lack of fiber in a tube feeding can cause:
    a. Constipation
    b. Nausea and vomiting
    c. Aspiration
    d. Diarrhea

3. The nursing activity most likely to prevent the clogging of a nasogastric feeding tube is:
    a. Attaching the tubing to suction after each feeding
    b. Flushing the tubing with water and clamping it after each feeding
    c. Clamping the tubing before all of the nourishment has drained
    d. Aspirate as much as possible from the tubing using a 50-ml syringe

4. When a patient is unable to eat or drink normally over a long period of time, which of the following would be the best alternative:
    a. Giving liquid nutrients through a tube leading from the nose to the stomach or intestine
    b. Giving solutions through tubing inserted into a peripheral vein
    c. Giving continuous tube feedings regulated via an electric feeding pump
    d. Giving feedings through a tube inserted through the skin and tissue of the abdomen

5. The process of removing poisonous substances through gastric intubation is called:
    a. Gavage
    b. Decompression
    c. Lavage
    d. Tamponade

6. Feeding-tube obstruction may occur if the formula is administered at a rate that is less than:
    a. 30 ml per hour
    b. 50 ml per hour
    c. 70 ml per hour
    d. 90 ml per hour

7. Which of the following feeding tubes is least likely to become obstructed:
    a. Nasogastric
    b. Nasointestinal
    c. Jejunostomy
    d. Gastrostomy

8. An advantage of the gastrostomy over other feeding tubes is:
    a. It has reduced potential for reflux and aspiration
    b. It is easy to insert
    c. It accommodates crushed medications
    d. It can remain in place for up to 4 weeks

9. Which of the following gastrointestinal tubes has the largest diameter:
    a. Sengstaken-Blakemore
    b. Levin
    c. Ewald
    d. Keofeed

10. Instillation of a large volume of liquid nourishment into the stomach in a fairly short time describes:
    a. A bolus feeding
    b. A cyclic feeding
    c. An intermittent feeding
    d. A continuous feeding

11. Most formulas used for tube feedings have a caloric value of:
    a. 1.5 to 2.0 kcal/ml
    b. 0.5 to 1.5 kcal/ml
    c. 0.5 to 2.0 kcal/ml
    d. 1.5 to 2.5 kcal/ml

12. Bolus formula feedings are the least desirable because they:
    a. Mimic the natural filling and emptying of the stomach
    b. Are given by gravity drip over an hour's time
    c. Are given during the late evening hours and during sleep
    d. Cause gastric reflux and increase the risk of aspiration

13. Gastric residual is best described as:
    a. A volume equal to 20% of the total volume of the previous hour's tube feeding
    b. The volume of liquid left in the stomach after allowing sufficient time for emptying to occur
    c. The volume of liquid from the stomach that empties into the small intestine
    d. The extra volume of formula from a feeding that will cause reflux and aspiration

14. Which of the following amounts represents an accurate estimate of the daily water requirement for adults receiving tube feedings:
    a. 30 ml/kg of weight
    b. 50 ml/kg of weight
    c. 70 ml/kg of weight
    d. 90 ml/kg of weight

15. Instilling a tube feeding rapidly can result in:
    a. Nausea and vomiting
    b. Constipation
    c. Weight loss
    d. Sore throat

TRUE OR FALSE QUESTIONS

Directions: For items 1 through 10, decide if the statement is true or false and mark T or F in the space provided.

1. _____ When preparing to give nourishment by gastric gavage, the nurse should prewarm the solution before administering it.
2. _____ A surgical opening into the stomach through the abdominal wall is called a gastrostomy.
3. _____ Nasogastric tube feedings are the method of choice when the patient requires an alternative to oral feeding for longer than a month.
4. _____ Incorrect nasogastric tube placement may cause aspiration.
5. _____ The distance from the earlobe to the xiphoid process approximates the length of tubing required for a nasogastric tube to reach the stomach.
6. _____ The least accurate test for determining the correct placement of a nasogastric tube is placing the end of the tube into a glass of water.
7. _____ The stylet for a small-diameter feeding tube should be reinserted while the tube is in the patient.
8. _____ The purpose for measuring gastric residual is to determine if the rate or volume is more than the physiological capacity of the patient.
9. _____ Intestinal decompression refers to the enteral feeding of patients who cannot tolerate oral nourishment.
10. _____ If the gastrostomy is accidentally extubated, the nurse may insert a mercury-weighted tube into the opening to maintain patency until re-intubation can be accomplished.

SHORT ANSWER QUESTIONS

Directions: Read each of the following statements and supply the word(s) necessary in the space provided.

1. Describe the approved methods for determining if a nasogastric tube is in the patient's stomach.
   a. _____
   b. _____
   c. _____

2. List the steps utilized for administering an intermittent feeding.
   a. _____
   b. _____
   c. _____
   d. _____
   e. _____
   f. _____
   g. _____
   h. _____
   i. _____
   j. _____
   k. _____
   l. _____

3. Describe four schedules for administering tube feedings.
   a. _____
   b. _____
   c. _____
   d. _____

4. Identify four purposes for gastrointestinal intubation.
   a. _____
   b. _____
   c. _____
   d. _____

CRITICAL THINKING EXERCISE

You are the nurse caring for a patient who has just had a nasogastric feeding tube removed. The patient tells you he is hungry and would like something to eat and drink. Identify nursing activities appropriate to supply nourishment and fluid for this client. State the rationale for your choices.

PERFORMANCE CHECKLIST

A. This section allows you to examine your techniques for caring for the patient who has gastrointestinal intubation.
1. Place a check mark in the "S" ("satisfactory") column if you used the recommended technique.
2. Place a check mark in the "N.I." ("needs improvement") column if you used some but not all of each recommended technique.

3. Place a check mark in the "U" ("unsatisfactory") column if you forgot to include that particular recommended technique.
4. The section for comment allows space to make notes about when further practice is indicated, what errors you made, suggestions that will improve your skills, and so on.

Recommended Technique	S.	N.I.	U.	Comments
Assist with introducing the tube into the stomach or duodenum, as ordered				
Connect the tube to the suctioning equipment and check it regularly for proper functioning				
Check the drainage regularly, note its character, and report anything unusual promptly				
Record intake and output accurately. See to it that the patient has nothing by mouth unless otherwise ordered				
Give oral hygiene frequently				
Position the patient comfortably, preferably in the low Fowler's position				
Offer throat care as needed				
Be prepared to assist with giving intravenous therapy to the patient				
Remove the tube properly after the therapy is discontinued				

(continued)

B. Examine your techniques when offering nourishment to a patient who has a gavage tube in place and complete the following form.

Recommended Technique	S.	N.I.	U	Comments
Warm nourishment if a large amount is to be given; do not warm nourishment given continuously				
Check to see that the gavage tube is properly placed in the stomach, using appropriate techniques				
Observe the health agency's policy about the next three techniques				
Check by aspiration to see whether previous feedings remain in the stomach				
Return aspirated stomach contents to the stomach; offer proportionately smaller amounts of new nourishment				
Offer no new nourishment if 100 ml or more were aspirated from the stomach, according to agency policy				
Pour nourishment into a syringe or funnel connected to the gavage tube				
Allow nourishment to enter the stomach slowly by gravity				
Do not allow the syringe or funnel to become empty while introducing the nourishment				
Flush the tube by introducing 1 to 2 ounces of water after the nourishment is given				
Clamp the tube between feedings				

CHAPTER 30

Urinary Elimination

SUMMARY

Elimination of excess water and wastes is a normal physiological function of the kidneys and urinary bladder. The urinary system eliminates excess fluid and toxic substances in a waste solution called urine. Illnesses and situations producing stress may interfere with this normal mechanism of elimination. When this function becomes impaired, it can be life-threatening.

This chapter reviews the process of urinary elimination and describes nursing skills for assessing and maintaining urinary elimination.

MATCHING QUESTIONS

Directions: For items 1 through 5, match the descriptions given in Part B with the types of incontinences in Part A.

Part A
1. _____ Stress incontinence
2. _____ Urge incontinence
3. _____ Reflex incontinence
4. _____ Functional incontinence
5. _____ Overflow incontinence

Part B
a. Control over urination is lost due to inaccessibility of a toilet or a compromised ability to use one
b. Loss of urine without any identifiable pattern or warning
c. Urine leaks because the bladder is not completely emptied and remains distended with retained urine
d. The need to void is perceived frequently with short-lived ability to sustain control of the flow
e. The loss of small amounts of urine during situations when intra-abdominal pressure rises
f. Spontaneous loss of urine when the bladder is stretched with urine, but without prior perception of a need to void

Directions: For items 6 through 10, match the nursing approaches in Part B with the types of incontinences in Part A.

6. _____ Stress incontinence
7. _____ Urge incontinence
8. _____ Functional incontinence
9. _____ Reflex incontinence
10. _____ Overflow incontinence

Part B
a. Modify clothing; facilitate access to a toilet, commode, or urinal; assist to a toilet according to a pre-planned schedule
b. Pelvic floor muscle strengthening; weight reduction
c. Hydration; adequate bowel elimination; maintain patency of catheter; credé the bladder
d. Absorbent undergarments; external catheter; indwelling catheter
e. Cutaneous triggering; straight intermittent catheterization
f. Maintain fluid intake of at least 2000 ml per day; omit bladder irritants, such as caffeine or alcohol; administer diuretics in the morning

MULTIPLE CHOICE QUESTIONS

Directions: For items 1 through 12, circle the letter that corresponds to the best answer for each question.

1. Urine is formed in the:
   a. Bladder
   b. Ureters
   c. Kidneys
   d. Urethra

2. The average adult will desire to empty his bladder when it contains:
   a. 100 to 150 ml of urine
   b. 200 to 300 ml of urine
   c. 250 to 400 ml of urine
   d. 400 to 500 ml of urine

189

3. The absence of urine is:
   a. Anuria
   b. Oliguria
   c. Polyuria
   d. Dysuria

4. The term that indicates the kidneys are not forming urine is:
   a. Oliguria
   b. Anuria
   c. Urinary retention
   d. Urinary suppression

5. Urine retained in the bladder after a patient voids is called:
   a. Overflow urine
   b. Residual urine
   c. Excess urine
   d. Secondary urine

6. Stress incontinence is best described as:
   a. The inability to retain urine within the bladder
   b. Increased abdominal pressure causes urine to be released
   c. The repeated awakening during the night to empty the bladder
   d. The voiding of small amounts at frequent intervals

7. The average amount of urine produced every 24 hours by healthy adults is:
   a. 1200 ml
   b. 1000 ml
   c. 1500 ml
   d. 500 ml

8. The term used to describe pus in the urine is:
   a. Glycosuria
   b. Hematuria
   c. Pyuria
   d. Albuminuria

9. For individuals who have stress incontinence, which of the following techniques is especially helpful to restore continence:
   a. The Credé maneuver
   b. The cutaneous triggering mechanism
   c. The Kegel exercises
   d. Intermittent straight catheterization

10. The nurse should propose the insertion of a catheter only when:
    a. The patient complains of bladder discomfort
    b. The benefits for the patient outweigh the risks
    c. The patient is embarrassed by his incontinence
    d. The family needs help in dealing with incontinence

11. The catheter that is intended to be inserted and withdrawn following its use for a temporary measure is:
    a. An indwelling catheter
    b. A Foley catheter
    c. A straight catheter
    d. A retention catheter

12. The most hazardous problem when external catheters are used:
    a. The blood supply to the tissues of the penis may be restricted
    b. The skin may break down due to the collection of moisture
    c. The catheter may not fit well and cause urine to leak out
    d. The catheter may not be kept as clean as is necessary by the patient

TRUE OR FALSE QUESTIONS

Directions: For items 1 through 12, decide if the statement is true or false and mark T or F in the space provided.

1. _____ Urine is transported from the kidneys to the bladder via the urethra.

2. _____ The synonym for urination is micturition.

3. _____ Oliguria refers to the absence of urine.

4. _____ Polyuria is the term for blood in the urine.

5. _____ Indwelling catheters should be irrigated routinely.

6. _____ Individuals with indwelling catheters should have an intake of 1000 to 1500 ml daily.

7. _____ Urinary tract infections are one of the most commonly acquired infections in patients who have indwelling catheters.

8. _____ The nurse must insist on sterile techniques when teaching a patient self-catheterization.

9. _____ The less skin that is exposed on the patient with a urinary diversion, the less the skin will be irritated.

10. _____ A midstream urine specimen is collected under sterile conditions.

11. _____ To ensure accuracy, the second voided specimen should be used when testing for sugar in the urine.

12. _____ Incontinent patients should be instructed to limit their fluid intake.

SHORT ANSWER QUESTIONS

Directions: Read each of the following statements and supply the word(s) necessary in the space provided.

1. List four actions that may be helpful when a male patient uses a urinal.
   a. _____
   b. _____
   c. _____
   d. _____

2. Identify eight suggestions that may be developed into a more specific plan for bladder retraining.
   a. _____ e. _____
   b. _____ f. _____
   c. _____ g. _____
   d. _____ h. _____

3. List six factors that influence the amount, contents, and characteristics of urine or its elimination.
   a. _____
   b. _____
   c. _____
   d. _____
   e. _____
   f. _____

4. List five nursing measures that can be utilized when the patient needs assistance with urination.
   a. _____
   b. _____
   c. _____
   d. _____
   e. _____

CRITICAL THINKING EXERCISES

1. Describe adjustments you make when prompting urinary elimination:
   a. When the patient is an infant or child

   b. When the patient is pregnant or in the early postpartal period

   c. When the patient is elderly

2. Plan a teaching program for a patient for whom you are caring and complete the following form.

Topic for Teaching	Points to Cover in the Teaching Program
Proper functioning of the urinary system, normal voiding, and normal urine	
Self-catheterization	
Home care, including common urine tests, of patients who have problems related to urinary elimination	
The collection of various types of specimens by the patient Single voided:	
Clean-catch midstream:	
24-hour specimen:	

PERFORMANCE CHECKLIST

A. This section allows you to examine your techniques for caring for the patient who requires assistance with urinary elimination.

1. Place a check mark in the "S" ("satisfactory") column if you used the recommended technique.
2. Place a check mark in the "N.I." ("needs improvement") column if you used some but not all of each recommended technique.
3. Place a check mark in the "U" ("unsatisfactory") column if you forgot to include that particular recommended technique.
4. The section for comment allows space to make notes about when further practice is indicated, what errors you made, suggestions that will improve your skills, and so on.

Recommended Technique	S	N.I.	U	Comments
Bring necessary equipment and supplies to the bedside; warm a metal bedpan, if indicated				
Piefold top bed linens back onto the patient and place the bedpan under the patient				
Roll the patient onto the bedpan if he cannot assist				
If the patient cannot lift or roll himself onto the bedpan, lift the patient under his lower back or obtain help to do so				
Place the urinal between slightly spread legs				
Raise the head of the bed slightly, if permitted				
Replace top linens, have the signal device and toilet tissue handy for the patient, and raise the bed siderails				
Provide a receptacle for toilet tissue when a specimen is needed and explain the reason to the patient				
Leave the patient for privacy or remain with the patient if indicated				
To remove the bedpan, piefold top linens and remove the bed pan or urinal as it was offered				
Cover the bedpan/urinal place it on a chair or at the foot of the bed; clean a helpless patient with toilet tissue				

(continued)

Recommended Technique	S	N.I.	U	Comments
Replace top bed linens and offer the patient equipment and supplies to wash his hands				
Collect a specimen, if required, while observing agency policy				

B. This section allows you to examine your techniques for inserting a catheter for a female patient.

Recommended Technique	S.	N.I.	U.	Comments
Assemble equipment, have the patient on a firm surface, and have good lighting available				
Position and drape the patient properly; clean the genital area, if necessary				
Set up the sterile field and don sterile gloves properly				
Lubricate the catheter about 3.75 to 5 centimeters (1.5 to 2 inches) without clogging the eyes of the catheter				
Open labia with thumb and fingers and expose the meatus well				
Clean the area at the meatus thoroughly and properly with the antiseptic solution of the agency's choice				
Insert the catheter 5 to 7.5 centimeters (2 to 3 inches) with a sterile gloved hand or pickup forceps				
Keep labia well separated until the urine flows freely				
Use no force to insert the catheter				
If the catheter meets resistance, try these techniques:				
Ask the patient to take deep breaths				
Rotate the catheter in place				
Ask the patient to wiggle the toes				
Withdraw the catheter and discontinue the procedure if continued resistance and discomfort are present				
Hold the catheter securely in place while the bladder empties and drain urine into a receptacle or specimen bottle				

Recommended Technique	S.	N.I.	U.	Comments
Withdraw the catheter slowly until urine barely drips and then withdraw the catheter completely				
Handle the urine specimen according to agency policy				
Work always with gentleness and while being particularly careful to observe surgical asepsis				

C. This section allows you to examine your techniques for inserting a catheter for a male patient.

Recommended Technique	S	N.I.	U	Comments
Lubricate the catheter generously for 15 to 17.5 centimeters (6 to 7 inches) without clogging the eyes of the catheter				
Lift the penis while cleaning at the meatus and down the shaft of the penis				
Pull the penis with gentle traction and slightly pinch the end of the penis to open the meatus				
Gently introduce the catheter while holding the penis almost vertical to the patient's body				
If resistance occurs, rotate the catheter in place, ask the patient to deep breathe, or place more traction on the penis				
If resistance is met in the area of the prostate gland, drop the penis a bit toward the patient's toes				
Clean under the foreskin and reduce it after catheterizing the uncircumcised male				
Observe techniques common to catheterizing men and women				

D. This section allows you to examine your techniques for caring for a patient with an indwelling catheter.

Recommended Technique	S	N.I.	U	Comments
Clean the perineal area and around the meatus at least twice a day and after each bowel movement				
Use soap and water or an antiseptic of the agency's choice for cleaning the perineal area				
See to it that the patient has a generous fluid intake				

(continued)

Recommended Technique	S	N. I.	U	Comments
Keep the tubing free of kinks				
Encourage and help the patient to be up and about as much as allowed				
Note the volume and characteristics of the urine and report anything unusual promptly				
Assist the patient who can take a shower or tub bath and manage his drainage system properly				
Teach the patient about the functioning and care of his drainage system				
Replace the indwelling catheter with a new one as indicated				
Empty the balloon completely before removing the indwelling catheter				
Continue to observe the patient for adverse signs due to having an indwelling catheter				
Continue to see to it that the patient's fluid intake is generous and that urinary output is carefully measured				

E. This section allows you to examine your techniques for irrigating an indwelling catheter.

Recommended Technique	S	N.I.	U	Comments
Gather necessary equipment, including sterile irrigating solution				
Clean the area well where the catheter and tubing join and disconnect them				
Protect the tubing with a sterile plug or a sponge moistened with antiseptic				
Inject about 60 ml of solution, or the prescribed amount, into the catheter				
Allow solution to flow back by gravity into a basin				
Milk catheter away from the bladder if the return is slow				
Reconnect the catheter and tubing and check for urine flow				
Note the amount of solution used for irrigating and the amount returned				
Use sterile and fresh irrigating solution; replace with fresh solution every 24 hours				

F. This section slows you to examine your technique for obtaining a clean-catch midstream urine specimen.

Recommended Technique	S	N.I.	U	Comments
From a Woman				
Gather the necessary equipment				
Position and drape the patient properly				
Don sterile gloves and separate the labia well with one hand				
Clean the area at the meatus properly with a cotton ball or gauze moistened with antiseptic				
Have the patient void about 30 ml into a basin while you hold the labia apart				
Ask the patient to void forcibly into a container while collecting the specimen				
Complete the collection of the specimen before the bladder is empty				
Allow the labia to fall into place and offer a bedpan to the patient to complete voiding				
From a Man				
Gather the necessary equipment				
Position the patient on his back or, if permitted, the patient may stand				
Don sterile gloves				
Retract the foreskin in an uncircumcised male and hold the foreskin back during the procedure				
Clean the area at the meatus and the shaft of the penis properly with an antiseptic				
Have the patient void about 30 ml into a basin while continuing to hold the foreskin back				
Ask the patient to void directly into the specimen container				
Complete the collection of the specimen before the bladder is empty				
Bring back the foreskin in an uncircumcised male and offer a urinal to the patient to finish voiding				

CHAPTER 31

Bowel Elimination

SUMMARY

Foods are digested, absorbed, and eliminated by structures in the gastrointestinal tract. Undigestible substances from food and some water are eliminated as stool, or feces. Efficient physiologic functioning requires that waste products be eliminated through the bowel. Generally, problems encountered are those of either too frequent elimination or those of infrequent elimination. If uncorrected, either situation may lead to death by altering the water and chemical balance in the body.

This chapter reviews the process of intestinal elimination and discusses measures to promote it.

MATCHING QUESTIONS

Directions: For items 1 through 8, match the types of constipation given in Part B with the contribution factors listed Part A. (Note: Items in Part B may be used more than one time.)

Part A
1. _____ Spinal cord compression
2. _____ Narcotic analgesia
3. _____ Decreased physical activity
4. _____ Partial intestinal obstruction
5. _____ Inadequate time for defecation
6. _____ Antidepressants
7. _____ Anticonvulsants
8. _____ Inadequate privacy

Part B
a. Primary or simple constipation
b. Secondary constipation
c. Iatrogenic constipation

MULTIPLE CHOICE QUESTIONS

Directions: For items 1 through 20, circle the letter that corresponds to the best answer for each question.

1. Of the following, which effect would a diet high in fiber and roughage have on normal intestinal elimination:
   a. The production of a smaller stool and the promotion of quicker passage
   b. The production of a larger stool and the promotion of quicker passage
   c. The production of a larger stool and the promotion of slower passage
   d. The production of a smaller stool and the promotion of slower passage

2. Constipation is best described as:
   a. A condition in which the individual is unable to have a daily bowel movement
   b. A condition in which there is a daily bowel movement of a small amount
   c. A condition in which the stool becomes dry and hard and requires straining for elimination
   d. A condition in which the stool is moist and soft and requires a laxative for elimination

3. A typical sysmptom of fecal impaction is:
   a. The frequent passing of flatus
   b. Liquid fecal seepage from the anus
   c. The passage of small, hard, and dry stool
   d. The lack of an urge to defecate

4. Of the following measures, which is used most often for a patient with a fecal impaction:
   a. A large-volume enema
   b. A hypertonic enema
   c. An oil retention enema
   d. A laxative or cathartic

199

5. The primary reason for using the digital method for patients with a fecal impaction is to:
   a. Relax the anal sphincter
   b. Lubricate the stool
   c. Stimulate the peristalsis
   d. Break up the fecal mass

6. An excessive amount of gas within the intestinal tract is called:
   a. Flatus
   b. Flatulence
   c. Tympanites
   d. Distention

7. The largest percentage of gas in the bowel comes from:
   a. Bacterial fermentation
   b. Spicy foods
   c. Swallowed air
   d. Diffusion from the bloodstream

8. Of the following measures, which one is most helpful for the relief of intestinal distention:
   a. Teach the patient to use Valsalva's maneuver
   b. Place the patient in a semisitting position
   c. Insert a rectal tube for twenty minutes
   d. Insert an intestinal tube through the nose

9. Diarrhea is best described by its:
   a. Odor
   b. Amount
   c. Frequency
   d. Consistency

10. Of the following, which foods would be the best for a patient who has had diarrhea:
    a. Applesauce, coffee, and lettuce
    b. Bananas, bran flakes, and orange juice
    c. Bananas, applesauce, and jello
    d. Fried chicken, tomatoes, and tea

11. An action that may help patients with fecal incontinence to establish a pattern of elimination is:
    a. Changing the diet to one of bland and nonirritating foods
    b. Consulting with the physician to give an enema every 2 to 3 days
    c. Consulting with the physician in order to give a laxative daily
    d. Teaching the patient to note sensations and ignore the urge

12. Following a large-volume enema, defecation usually occurs within:
    a. 5 to 15 minutes
    b. 10 to 20 minutes
    c. 15 to 25 minutes
    d. 20 to 30 minutes

13. Tap water enemas that are repeated one after the other can:
    a. Irritate the mucous membrane
    b. Change elimination habits
    c. Result in fluid imbalances
    d. Cause loss of peristalsis

14. Hypertonic enema solutions act by:
    a. Preventing water absorption
    b. Softening the stool
    c. Breaking up fecal impactions
    d. The principle of osmosis

15. The recommended position for the administration of a hypertonic solution enema is:
    a. Left side lying
    b. Right side lying
    c. Knee-chest
    d. Prone

16. The primary purpose of an oil retention enema is to:
    a. Lubricate and soften the stool
    b. Increase the fluid in the bowel
    c. Break up fecal impactions
    d. Increase peristalsis

17. One of the biggest challenges in ostomy care is:
    a. Controlling the embarrassment of the patient
    b. Regulating the time of elimination for the patient
    c. Regulating the odor from the appliance for the patient
    d. Preventing skin breakdown for the patient

18. The nurse should assess the intestinal elimination patterns accurately for the elderly patient because:
    a. They are easily confused about their patterns of elimination
    b. They will need to be taught bowel retraining before discharge
    c. They usually have poor knowledge regarding their need for fecal elimination
    d. They may be very bowel conscious and report problems of constipation erroneously

19. An important teaching responsibility for nurses regarding intestinal elimination is:
    a. Explaining the different types of laxatives to patients
    b. Teaching the proper use and dangers of abuse regarding enemas and laxatives
    c. Explaining the different types and uses of over-the-counter enema preparations
    d. Explaining that it is important to have daily intestinal elimination

20. When is the gastrocolic reflex most active:
    a. Prior to defecation
    b. While sleeping
    c. After eating
    d. During digestion

TRUE OR FALSE QUESTIONS

Directions: For items 1 through 12, decide if the statement is true or false and mark T or F in the space provided.

1. _____ The internal anal sphincter is under voluntary control.
2. _____ Nervous tension may cause abdominal cramping and diarrhea.
3. _____ Constipation is described as the inability to have a daily intestinal elimination.
4. _____ Routine use of laxatives, enemas, or suppositories is often the cause of constipation.
5. _____ The amount of water retained in the stool is dependent upon the undigestible fiber content of the diet.
6. _____ A patient with fecal impaction may expel liquid stool around the impacted mass.
7. _____ Eating spicy foods increases the volume of gas in the intestinal tract and lengthens the transit time.
8. _____ Diarrhea is described as frequent intestinal elimination.
9. _____ A hypertonic enema solution causes fluids to move from the feces into the bowel, causing peristalsis.
10. _____ An ileostomy is an opening into the large intestine.
11. _____ A continent ostomy is also referred to as a Kock pouch.
12. _____ The normal aging processes tend to predispose a person to constipation.

SHORT ANSWER QUESTIONS

Directions: Read each of the following statements and supply the word(s) necessary in the space provided.

1. List the conditions that predispose a person to form greater amounts of gas or interfere with its absorption.

   _____
   _____
   _____
   _____

2. List the chief characteristics of constipation.

   _____
   _____
   _____

3. Identify causes of diarrhea as suggested in this chapter.

   _____
   _____
   _____

4. Identify nursing measures suggested in this chapter for relieving the effects of diarrhea.

   _____
   _____
   _____

5. Identify causes of fecal incontinence as suggested in this chapter.

   _____
   _____
   _____

CRITICAL THINKING EXERCISES

1. Visit a pharmacy and make a list of several of the over-the-counter medications available for alleviating constipation or diarrhea. Choose three medications in either category and compare their actions, side effects and cautions. Write a teaching plan that you could use for a patient who chooses self-medication to relieve their problem. You may want to share your plan with your instructor and fellow students.

2. Prepare a teaching plan for a patient experiencing the following alterations in bowel elimination:

Topic for Teaching	Points to Cover in a Teaching Program
The abuse of enemas and laxatives	
Self-administering a cleansing enema when using a hypertonic solution and when using a large volume of solution	
Relieving common problems related to elimination:	
Constipation	
Diarrhea	
Fecal incontinence	
Abdominal distention	
Fecal impaction	
Self-care of a colostomy	
Self-care of an ileostomy	
The collection of a stool specimen by a patient	

PERFORMANCE CHECKLIST

A. This section allows you to examine your techniques for caring for the patient who requires a rectal tube.

1. Place a check mark in the "S" ("satisfactory") column if you used the recommended technique.
2. Place a check mark in the "N.I." ("needs improvement") column if you used some but not all of each recommended technique.

3. Place a check mark in the "U" ("unsatisfactory") column if you forgot to include that particular recommended technique.
4. The section for comment allows space to make notes about when further practice is indicated, what errors you made, suggestions that will improve your skills, and so on.

Recommended Technique	S	N.I.	U	Comments
Assemble necessary equipment, wash hands				
Position and drape the patient properly				
Lubricate the rectal tube				
Separate the buttocks well and insert the tube about 10 cm (4 inches)				
Provide for a proper method to collect discharge passed through the rectal tube				
Leave the rectal tube in place for about 20 minutes				
Reinsert the tube every 2 to 3 hours as necessary until relief from abdominal distention occurs				

B. This section allows you to examine your techniques for inserting a rectal suppository.

Recommended Technique	S	N.I.	U	Comments
Assemble necessary equipment, wash hands				
Position and drape the patient properly				
Don a glove or finger cot and separate the buttocks well				
Insert the suppository through the anus and beyond the internal sphincter				
Explain to the patient that she is to retain the suppository until she has a strong urge to defecate				
Assist the patient to walk about, if she is permitted to do so, while retaining the suppository				

(continued)

C. This section allows you to examine your techniques for administering a cleansing enema.

Recommended Technique	S	N.I.	U	Comments
Assemble necessary equipment and supplies				
Have a bedpan, commode, or bathroom ready for the patient's use, wash hands				
Position and drape the patient properly, put on gloves				
Lubricate about 5 to 7.5 centimeters (2 to 3 inches) of the rectal tube and allow solution to fill the tubing				
Lift the buttocks to expose the anus and slowly insert the tube 7.5 to 10 centimeters (3 to 4 inches) at an angle pointing to the umbilicus				
Use various techniques if resistance is met while inserting the rectal tube:				
Permit a little solution to enter, withdraw the tube a bit, and continue to insert the tube				
Have the patient take several deep breaths				
Place warm compresses over the anal area				
Do not force entry of the tube or place the solution more than 50 centimeters (20 inches) above the level of the patient's anus				
Intruduce the solution slowly over a period of 5 to 10 minutes				
To reduce the urge to defecate, have the patient take panting breaths, slow flow rate, and/or place pressure on anus				
Help the patient retain the solution until a strong urge to defecate is present				
Assist the patient as necessary to use a bedpan, commode, or a bathroom				
Note the character of the stool and leave the patient clean and comfortable				
Care for the equipment according to agency policy				
If a patient has an erection, handle the situation in a matter-of-fact manner				

D. This section allows you to examine your techniques for caring for a patient with a colostomy.

Recommended Technique	S	N.I.	U	Comments
Have patient's skin clean and free of soap and pat the area dry before applying a bag or dressing to the ostomy				
Wash hands, put on gloves				
Protect the skin around the stoma with a preparation of agency's choice, as indicated				
Put the appliance on the patient's stoma according to manufacturer's directions				
Observe methods and teach the patient how to control odors and how to clean and deodorize the appliance				
Teach the patient how his ostomy functions and where he can obtain help if it becomes necessary				
Offer the patient necessary support as he learns to live with his ostomy				

E. This section allows you to examine your techniques for irrigating a colostomy.

Recommended Technique	S	N.I.	U	Comments
Assemble necessary equipment; wash hands; put on gloves				
Position and drape the patient properly				
Fill the tubing and cone with irrigating solution				
Remove dressings from the stoma or the appliance and place the irrigating sleeve over the stoma				
Lubricate the irrigating cone				
Introduce the cone into the stoma gently while following the contour of the colon				
Do not force the cone; discontinue the preocedure if undue resistance is met				
After cone is in place, allow solution to enter the colon slowly				
Hold the solution container no more than about 30 centimeters (12 inches) above the patient's pelvis				

(continued)

Recommended Technique	S	N.I.	U	Comments
Shut off the solution flow temporarily if the patient complains of cramping				
After the solution is introduced, remove the cone and close the top of the irrigating sleeve				
Prepare to receive the return in a bedpan, commode, or toilet				
When the return has stopped, care for the stoma properly				

CHAPTER 32

Oral Medications

SUMMARY

Medications, or drugs, are physiologic agents used to treat pathologic conditions. They are substances that chemically change body functions when taken by an individual. The focus of this chapter is the nurse's responsibility for the safe preparation and administration of oral agents.

MATCHING QUESTIONS

Directions: For items 1 through 6, match the abbreviations in Part B with the meanings in Part A.

Part A

1. _____ Immediately
2. _____ Every other day
3. _____ Every day
4. _____ Every 4 hours
5. _____ Twice a day
6. _____ Four times a day

Part B
   a. t.i.d.
   b. q.i.d.
   c. q.o.d.
   d. stat
   e. q.h.
   f. q.d.
   g. b.i.d.
   h. q.4h.

Directions: For items 7 through 10, match the method of Administration in Part B with the route in Part A.

Part A

7. _____ Oral
8. _____ Topical
9. _____ Inhalant
10. _____ Parenteral.

Part B
   a. Injection
   b. Aerosol
   c. Swallowing
   d. Application to skin

MULTIPLE CHOICE QUESTIONS

Directions: For items 1 through 12, circle the letter that corresponds to the best answer for each question.

1. The trade or proprietary name for a drug refers to:
   a. The drug's chemical makeup
   b. The manufacturer's name
   c. The drug's generic name
   d. The action of the drug

2. A medication order should never be implemented if the nurse:
   a. Does not know the physician
   b. Does not know the patient's history
   c. Questions any part of the order
   d. Did not witness the writing of the order

3. Most health agencies check narcotic supplies:
   a. Once each day by two nurses
   b. Twice each day by a nurse and a pharmacist
   c. At the change of each shift by two nurses
   d. Three times a day by two pharmacists

4. To ensure that medications are prepared and administered correctly, the nurse should:
   a. Use the patient's rights
   b. Use the FIVE RIGHTS
   c. Give the medication only when requested
   d. Give the medication without question

5. The minimum number of times the nurse should check the label when preparing to give medications is:
   a. Two times
   b. Three times
   c. Four times
   d. Five times

6. If a patient is on the telephone when the nurse delivers his medication, the correct procedure would be to:
   a. Return the medication to a safe place and record it as refused
   b. Leave it with the patient and tell him to take it when he finishes
   c. Ask another nurse to give the medication when he is finished
   d. Wait until he excuses himself and have him take the medication

7. If Mr. S. states that the pill he has been receiving is a different color, the correct procedure for the nurse would be to:
   a. Explain that she will check the situation and return later
   b. Explain that the pharmacy often substitutes and this is the same
   c. Tell Mr. S that he is probably confused and the medication is correct
   d. Explain that this is the right medication because the physician ordered it

8. The first action to take when a medication error takes place is:
   a. Call the physician
   b. Call the supervisor
   c. Complete an incident report
   d. Check the patient

9. Enteric-coated tablets are supposed to dissolve in the:
   a. Esophagus
   b. Stomach
   c. Small intestine
   d. Large intestine

10. Of the following, which is the main reason the nurse should stay with the patient until the oral medication is swallowed:
    a. All liquid that is ingested is considered part of the fluid intake
    b. An unopened unit dose drug can be saved if the patient refuses it
    c. The nurse is responsible for documenting that the drug was taken
    d. The nurse is the only one who can give the patient medications

11. When administering medication via nasogastric tubing that is being used for suction, clamp the tube for at least:
    a. One hour prior to medication administration to prevent complications
    b. One-half hour after instilling medication to allow for absorption
    c. One-and one-half hours after instilling medication to allow for absorption
    d. One-half hour prior to medication administration to prevent complications

12. Elderly patients may have an increased risk of adverse side effects and toxicity to drugs because of:
    a. Poor circulation
    b. Decreased mobility
    c. Decreased gastrointestinal motility
    d. Decreased mental capacity

TRUE OR FALSE QUESTIONS

Directions: For items 1 through 12, decide if the statement is true or false and mark T or F in the space provided.

1. _____ Safe practice is to follow only a written order for medications.

2. _____ The nurse may delegate the responsibility of checking and transcribing medication orders to clerical personnel.

3. _____ The proprietary name of a drug is usually descriptive of the drug's chemical structure.

4. _____ The nurse is expected to question any medication order that does not contain all of its parts.

5. _____ A drug that is ordered to be given four times a day is routinely scheduled at 8 a.m., 12 noon, 4 p.m., and 8 p.m.

6. _____ State law requires that a record be kept for each narcotic that is administered.

7. _____ The patient has a right to refuse a medication.

8. _____ The patient's right to refuse a medication is one of the FIVE RIGHTS.

9. _____ An incident report must be filed with the patient's permanent record if the nurse commits a medication error.

10. _____ Medications that are not given because the patient is off the nursing unit for x-ray studies are considered errors.

11. _____ Medications may be mixed and administered along with continuous tube feedings.

12. _____ Enteric-coated tablets may be crushed and mixed with water prior to administration through nasogastric tubing.

SHORT ANSWER QUESTIONS

Directions: Read each of the following statements and supply the word(s) necessary in the space provided.

1. List the parts of a complete medication order.

    _____

    _____

    _____

2. Identify items of information the nurse should know about the patient before administering medications.

    _____

    _____

    _____

3. List the FIVE RIGHTS pertaining to administering medications.

    _____

    _____

    _____

4. Identify the steps that should be carried out prior to preparing drugs that will be administered to a patient as suggested in this chapter.

    _____

    _____

    _____

5. Identify guidelines, the nurse should follow when preparing medications for administration as suggested in this chapter.

    _____

    _____

    _____

CRITICAL THINKING EXERCISES

The following are practice situations for calculating medication dosages. Read each statement carefully, state the formula, and compute the correct dosage for each.

1. 60 mg of a drug is ordered. It is supplied in tablets containing 20 mg per tablet. How many tablets should be administered?

2. 50 mg of a drug is ordered. It is supplied in tablets containing 100 mg per tablet. How many tablets should be administered?

3. 250 mg of a drug is ordered, It is supplied in tablets of 0.5 g per tablet. How many tablets should be administered?

4. 1 g of a drug is ordered. It is supplied in tablets of 500 mg per tablet. How many tablets should be administered?

5. A dosage of gr 1/2 is ordered. It is supplied in a dosage of 60 mg per tablet. How many tablets should be administered?

PERFORMANCE CHECKLIST

A. This section allows you to examine your techniques for preparing and administering medication.
1. Place a check mark in the "S" ("satisfactory") column if you used the recommended technique.
2. Place a check mark in the "N.I." ("needs improvement") column if you used some but not all of each recommended technique.

3. Place a check mark in the "U" ("unsatisfactory") column if you forgot to include that particular recommended technique.
4. The section for comment allows space to make notes about when further practice is indicated, what errors you made, suggestions that will improve your skills, and so on.

Recommended Technique	S	N.I.	U	Comments
Know the patient's medication history				
Know the patient's diagnosis, plan of care, and expected results of medication therapy				
Know about each medication to be administered:				
Common average dosage				
Hoped for and undesirable effects				
Reasons for its use Symptoms of toxicity				
Common route of administration				
Time your work so that medications are given as near the specified time as possible				
Check the medication order carefully according to agency policy				
Be suspicious when a dosage has been increased or decreased markedly				
Follow accepted abbreviations only				
Prepare the medications while using a good light and work alone				
Check the label on the drug container three times when using a stock supply of the drug				
Do not use medications from containers when the label is difficult to read; do not guess				
Do not return medications to a container or transfer drugs from one container to another				

(continued)

Recommended Technique	S	N.I.	U	Comments
Do not use a medication that has a sediment, has a change of color, or appears cloudy				
Prepare medications in the order in which they will be given and arrange them accordingly for transporting				
Transport the medications to the patient carefully and safely, using methods recommended by the agency				
Protect needle for injecting drugs to prevent contamination according to agency policy				
Do not leave medications out of sight while administering drugs to patients				
Identify patients carefully and accurately before administering medications				
Do not give a medication if the patient says he is allergic to it or if signs/symptoms suggest an unfavorable reaction				
Check further if the patient believes he is receiving a new or different medication that has not been ordered				
Report immediately when a patient refuses a medication or has an unfavorable reaction to it in case of error, check the patient's condition and report the error promptly				
Do not give medications prepared by other persons				
Observe the FIVE RIGHTS of preparing and giving medications: the right drug, dose, route, time, and patient				

B. This section allows you to examine your techniques for administering oral medications.

Recommended Technique	S	N.I.	U	Comments
Pour capsules or tablets into the cap of the container				
Open prepackaged single-dose medications at the patient's bedside				
Pour liquids from a bottle opposite the label and into an appropriate measuring device				
Use an extractor properly when one is available				

Recommended Technique	S	N.I.	U	Comments
Read the amount of liquid medication at the bottom of the meniscus				
Have medications for the same patient in separate containers and offer them to the patient separately				
Offer fluids generously for certain medications or to swallow capsules or pills, unless contraindicated				
Offer no fluids with a liquid used to control a cough				
Use a drinking tube when medications are likely to stain or damage the teeth				
Chill a medication that has an objectionable taste, disguise it, or use ice chips as necessary				
Stay with the patient until all medications are swallowed and leave no medications at the patient's bedside				

C. This section allows you to examine your techniques for administering medications through a nasogastric tube.

Recommended Technique	S	N.I.	U	Comments
Prepare the prescribed medication by dissolving crushed tablets or capsule contents in about 30 ml of warm water				
Assemble necessary equipment and the medication at the patient's bedside				
Drape patient properly				
Correctly test for placement of the nasogastric tube				
Attach syringe barrel or funnel to the clamped tube				
Pour medication in solution into the syringe barrel or funnel				
Open the clamp and allow the medication to enter the stomach				
Add 30 to 50 ml of water to flush the tube before the syringe or funnel is completely empty				
After all solution has entered, remove the barrel or funnel and clamp the tube				
Have the patient remain in a sitting position or on his right side with the head slightly elevated				
If the medication is to act on stomach mucosa, have the patient lie on his left side				

CHAPTER 33

Topical and Inhalant Medications

SUMMARY

Medications may be given by several routes other than oral. The focus of this chapter is the nurse's responsibility for the safe preparation and administration of topical and inhalant medications.

MATCHING QUESTIONS

Directions: For items 1 through 5, match the locations in Part B with the routes of administration in Part A.

Part A

1. _____ Cutaneous
2. _____ Sublingual
3. _____ Buccal
4. _____ Otic
5. _____ Ophthalmic

Part B

a. Between the cheek and gum
b. Within the ear
c. Under the tongue
d. Within the eye
e. To the skin

MULTIPLE CHOICE QUESTIONS

Directions: For items 1 through 10, circle the letter that corresponds to the best answer for each question.

1. To ensure good absorption when applying an inunction, the nurse should first:
   a. Cleanse the area with soap or detergent and water
   b. Warm the inunction to body temperature
   c. Cleanse the skin with an antiseptic solution
   d. Apply heat to the area for several minutes

2. Of the following, which is contraindicated when applying nitroglycerin to the skin:
   a. Remove any previous application from the patient's skin
   b. Apply the ointment on a clean, non-hairy surface of the skin
   c. Rub the ointment into the patient's skin with your fingers
   d. Cover the area with a square of plastic and tape the sides

3. When giving eardrops to an adult, the ear should be gently pulled:
   a. Upward and forward
   b. Upward and backward
   c. Downward and forward
   d. Downward and backward

4. When giving eardrops to a child, the ear should be gently pulled:
   a. Upward and forward
   b. Upward and backward
   c. Downward and forward
   d. Downward and backward

5. The term for a medication that is administered under the tongue is:
   a. Buccal
   b. Sublingual
   c. Subcutaneous
   d. Transdermal

6. The position of choice when inserting a vaginal medication is:
   a. Sim's position
   b. Knee-chest position
   c. Dorsal recumbent position
   d. Horizontal recumbent position

7. The mucous membrane of the eye is called the:
   a. Conjunctiva
   b. Sclera
   c. Cornea
   d. Retina

8. If medication must be instilled in both ears, it is appropriate to wait how long between applications:
   a. 5 minutes
   b. 10 minutes
   c. 15 minutes
   d. 20 minutes

9. Chewing, swallowing, smoking, eating, and drinking are contraindicated when which of the following medications are given?
   a. Otic
   b. Ophthalmic
   c. Inunction
   d. Buccal

10. When administering vaginal medications, the applicator is usually inserted into the vagina approximately:
    a. 1 to 2 inches
    b. 2 to 4 inches
    c. 3 to 5 inches
    d. 5 to 10 inches

TRUE OR FALSE QUESTIONS

Directions: For items 1 through 9, decide if the statement is true or false and mark T or F in the space provided.

1. _____   Topically applied drugs have only a local effect.
2. _____   It is often necessary to shave body hair prior to applying a transdermal patch.
3. _____   Solutions, ointments, and equipment used to administer eye medications should be sterile.
4. _____   The lack of subcutaneous fat in older adults may cause a topical medication to be absorbed more rapidly than in a younger adult.
5. _____   Bronchodilating drugs cause bradycardia and hypotension in susceptible individuals.
6. _____   The rebound effect is a phenomenon characterized by rapid swelling of nasal mucosa.
7. _____   Intense itching, redness with excoriation, and burning on urination are common signs and symptoms of vaginal yeast infections.

8. _____   The inhalant route is used for medication administration because the lungs provide a massive area of tissue from which drugs may be absorbed.
9. _____   Cutaneous applications are medications that are incorporated into a transporting agent.

SHORT ANSWER QUESTIONS

Directions: Read each of the following statements and supply the word(s) necessary in the space provided.

1. List the guidelines for giving an inunction.
   _____
   _____
   _____

2. List the guidelines for applying nitroglycerin ointment.
   _____
   _____
   _____

3. List the common routes of topical administration for drugs.
   _____
   _____
   _____

4. Identify six items necessary for patient teaching for self-administration of vaginal medications.
   _____
   _____
   _____

CRITICAL THINKING EXERCISE

Describe the current system for distributing medications to patients in the hospital where you care for patients. What are the checks and balances in this system to protect the patient and the nurse from medication errors?

PERFORMANCE CHECKLIST

A. This section allows you to examine your techniques for administering medications transdermally.
1. Place a check mark in the "S" ("satisfactory") column if you used the recommended technique.
2. Place a check mark in the "N.I." ("needs improvement") column if you used some but not all of each recommended technique.
3. Place a check mark in the "U" ("unsatisfactory") column if you forgot to include that particular recommended technique.
4. The section for comment allows space to make notes about when further practice is indicated, what errors you made, suggestions that will improve your skills, and so on.

Recommended Technique	S	N.I.	U	Comments
When an Ointment Dispensed from a Tube is Used				
Squeeze the prescribed amount onto the manufacturer's application paper				
Place the application paper on a clean, non-hairy area on the chest wall or upper arm				
Secure the application paper and cover it appropriately with plastic				
Check the patient's blood pressure 30 minutes after applying nitroglycerin				
Notify proper personnel when a fall in blood pressure and a rise in pulse rate do not occur when nitroglycerin is given				
Rotate sites on which ointment is placed				
Be careful not to get ointment on your own skin				
When a Disk of Ointment Is Used				
Follow above techniques, except for the following differences:				
Apply a disk according to directions, usually behind the patient's ear				
Monitor the patient appropriately, depending on the medication				

(continued)

B. This section allows you to examine your techniques for administering a medication topically.

Recommended Technique	S	N.I.	U	Comments
Apply a preparation to the skin				
Instill a solution into the eyes				
Instill a solution into the ears				
Use throat applications				
Instill a medication into the vagina				

C. This section allows you to examine your technique for administering a nasal medication.

Recommended Technique	S	N.I.	U	Comments
Compare the MAR with the written medical order				
Wash your hands				
Identify the patient				
Position the patient in a sitting position or place a rolled towel under the neck				
Remove the cap from the medication dropper				
Aim the tip of the dropper toward the nares				
Squeeze the rubber portion to give the correct number of drops				
Instruct the patient to breathe through the mouth as the drops are instilled				
If the Drug Is a Spray Form				
Place the tip of the container just inside the nostril				
Occlude the opposite nostril				
Instruct the patient to inhale as the spray is released				
Repeat on the opposite side as required				
Advise the patient to remain in the sitting position for about 5 minutes				
Recap and replace the container where medications are stored				
Document the administration on the MAR				

D. This section allows you to examine your technique for administering eye medications.

Recommended Technique	S	N.I.	U	Comments
Compare the MAR with the written medical order				
Warm eye drops and ointments by holding them in the hands				
Wash your hands				
Position the patient supine or sitting with head tilted back				
Cleanse the lids and lashes as needed				
Instruct the patient to look toward the ceiling				
Make a pouch in the lower lid by pulling the skin over the bony orbit downward				
Bring the medication container to the eye from below the patient's line of vision				
Instill the prescribed number of drops				
Instruct the patient to close the eyes and blink gently				
Wipe away excess with a clean tissue				
Document medication administration on the MAR				

E. This section allows you to examine your technique for teaching the patient how to use a metered dose inhaler.

Recommended Technique	S	N.I.	U	Comments
Instruct the Patient to Do the Following				
Attach the stem of the canister into the hole of the mouthpiece				
Shake the canister to distribute the drug within the pressurized chamber				
Exhale slowly through pursed lips				
Seal lips around the mouthpiece				
Compress the canister; slowly inhale				
Release the pressure on the canister; continue inhaling				
Withdraw the mouthpiece from the mouth				
Hold your breath a few seconds				
Exhale slowly through pursed lips				

Parenteral Medications

SUMMARY

The parenteral route (route of drug administration other than oral or through the gastrointestinal tract) commonly is used to refer to medications given by injection. This chapter discusses the techniques for administering injections. Preparation and administration follow the principles of asepsis and infection control.

MATCHING QUESTIONS

Directions: For items 1 through 4, match the injection routes in Part B with the injection sites in Part A.

Part A

1. _____   Inner aspect of the forearm
2. _____   Upper arm, thigh, abdomen, and back
3. _____   Dorsogluteal, vastus lateralis, and deltoid
4. _____   Blood vessels

Part B

a. intramuscular
b. subcutaneous
c. intravenous
d. intradermal

MULTIPLE CHOICE QUESTIONS

Directions: For items 1 through 12, circle the letter that corresponds to the best answer for each question.

1. When combining drugs from two multiple-dose vials, which procedure best ensures that the second vial will not be contaminated with medication from the first vial:
   a. Change the needle before inserting it into the second vial
   b. Cleanse the rubber stopper of each vial with an antiseptic
   c. Withdraw the exact amount of medication from the first vial
   d. Withdraw the exact amount of medication from the second vial

2. The common site for giving intramuscular injections into the gluteus maximus is the:
   a. Rectus femoris site
   b. Vastus lateralis site
   c. Dorsogluteal site
   d. Ventrogluteal site

3. The common site for giving intramuscular injections into the anterior aspect of the thigh is the:
   a. Rectus femoris site
   b. Vastus lateralis site
   c. Dorsogluteal site
   d. Ventrogluteal site

4. The preferred intramuscular injection site for infants is the:
   a. Vastus lateralis site
   b. Rectus femoris site
   c. Dorsogluteal site
   d. Ventrogluteal site

5. Intramuscular injections into the deltoid muscle should be limited to:
   a. 2.5 ml of solution
   b. 2 ml of solution
   c. 1 ml of solution
   d. 0.5 ml of solution

6. An accepted method for determining the dorsog-luteal site for an intramuscular injection is to:
   a. Palpate the greater trochanter at the head of the femur, the anterior superior iliac spine, and the iliac crest
   b. Palpate the posterior iliac spine and the greater trochanter and draw an imaginary line between the landmarks
   c. Divide the thigh into thirds using the hands and inject the medication into the middle third
   d. Place the palm of the hand on the greater trochanter and the index finger on the anterior superior iliac spine

7. The primary reason for using the Z-track technique when giving an intramuscular medication is to help:
   a. Avoid striking a major nerve
   b. Seal off the medication in the muscle
   c. Hasten the absorption of the medication
   d. Decrease the discomfort of the injection

8. The needle size for subcutaneous injections is usually:
   a. 20 gauge, 1/2 to 5/8 inch
   b. 21 gauge, 1/2 to 5/8 inch
   c. 22 gauge, 1/2 to 5/8 inch
   d. 25 gauge, 1/2 to 5/8 inch

9. The strength of insulin prepared by pharmaceutical companies is:
   a. 200 units of insulin per 1 ml
   b. 100 units of insulin per 1 ml
   c. 50 units of insulin per 1 ml
   d. 25 units of insulin per 1 ml

10. A primary concern when giving heparin subcuta-neously is to prevent:
    a. Bleeding and bruising
    b. Pain and bruising
    c. Pain and bleeding
    d. Injecting a vein

11. The angle of the syringe and needle for intradermal injections is:
    a. 90 degrees
    b. 45 to 90 degrees
    c. 10 to 45 degrees
    d. 10 to 15 degrees

12. Humulin N is an example of an insulin that is:
    a. Long acting
    b. Intermediate acting
    c. Short acting
    d. Ultra-fast acting

TRUE OR FALSE QUESTIONS

Directions: For items 1 through 11, decide if the statement is true or false and mark T or F in the space provided.

1. _____ Parenteral refers to all oral medications.
2. _____ The smaller the number of the gauge, the larger the lumen of the needle.
3. _____ When combining medications from sin-gle-dose and multiple-dose vials, the medication should be withdrawn from the single-dose vials first.
4. _____ The terms vial and ampule are synonymous.
5. _____ When administering an intramuscular medication, the needle should be intro-duced slowly to prevent tissue damage.
6. _____ The advantage of prefilled medication cartridges for injection is that the dosage is always correct.
7. _____ Prefilled cartridges are often intended for multiple-dose use and should be checked carefully.
8. _____ When planning to give an injection via the Z-track technique, it is not necessary to change the needle after aspirating the medication into the syringe.
9. _____ Subcutaneous medications may be given at a 90 degree angle.
10. _____ It is a common practice for one nurse to check the insulin preparation of another nurse.
11. _____ When giving heparin subcutaneously, the plunger of the syringe must be aspirated to make certain the needle is not in a blood vessel.

SHORT ANSWER QUESTIONS

Directions: Read each of the following statements and supply the word(s) necessary in the space provided.

1. Identify four criteria for selecting the appropriate syringe and needle for the administration of par-enteral medications.
   a. _____
   b. _____
   c. _____
   d. _____

2. Identify four postneedle-stick activities that are recommended to protect your health.

   a. _____

   b. _____

   c. _____

   d. _____

Describe alternative techniques the nurse could use to reduce discomfort associated with injections. State the rationale for their use.

PERFORMANCE CHECKLIST

A. This section allows you to examine your techniques for removing medications from vials and ampules.
1. Place a check mark in the "S" ("satisfactory") column if you used the recommended technique.
2. Place a check mark in the "N.I." ("needs improvement") column if you used some but not all of each recommended technique.

3. Place a check mark in the "U" ("unsatisfactory") column if you forgot to include that particular recommended technique.
4. The section for comment allows space to make notes about when further practice is indicated, what errors you made, suggestions that will improve your skills, and so on.

Recommended Technique	S	N.I.	U	Comments
From a Vial				
Remove the soft metal cover on the vial				
Cleanse the exposed rubber cap with a pledget moistened with an antiseptic				
Fill the syringe with the same amount of air as the amount of solution to be withdrawn				
Insert the needle into the cap at a slight angle and withdraw the desired amount of solution				
Hold the vial straight and at eye level while withdrawing solution				
Withdraw the needle from the vial and prepare to administer the medication				
From an Ampule				
Tap the stem of the ampule until all of the medication is in the well of the ampule				
Cleanse the area where the ampule will be broken with a pledget moistened with antiseptic				
Hold the ampule in one hand and protect the fingers of the other hand with a dry pledget				
Break off the stem of the ampule with the fingers				
Insert the needle into the opened ampule, being careful not to touch the edges of the glass				

(continued)

Recommended Technique	S	N.I.	U	Comments
Remove the medication from the ampule by pulling back on the plunger of the syringe				
Remove the needle without touching the edges of the ampule and discard the ampule				

B. This section allows you to examine your techniques for administering intramuscular and subcutaneous injections.

Recommended Technique	S	N.I.	U	Comments
Intramuscular Injection				
Select proper equipment and supplies and, unless syringe is prefilled, accurately fill the syringe with the drug				
Demonstrate how to locate the proper site for injecting into dorsogluteal, ventrogluteal, vastus lateralis, rectus femoris, and deltoid muscles				
Use appropriate techniques to reduce discomfort before giving an injection				
Select an appropriate site for injecting the medication mid cleanse the area properly				
Press the tissue down firmly and quickly thrust the needle for most of its length into the muscle tissue				
Aspirate to see whether the needle is in a vein; if it is, follow agency policy:				
Remove needle, replace it, and select a new site				
Withdraw needle slightly, move it laterally a bit, and, if no blood is then aspirated, inject the medication				
Discard the needle, syringe, and medication, and prepare fresh medication for injection into another site				
If the needle is not in a vein, inject the medication slowly, followed by the air bubble				
Withdraw the needle quickly while applying pressure against the injection site				
Massage the area for a minute or two, unless the manufacturer recommends otherwise				

Recommended Technique	S	N.I.	U	Comments
Z-Track Technique				
Select and prepare the site where the medication is to be injected				
Grasp the patient's muscle with your non-dominant hand near the site where the injection is to be made				
Pull the skin and underlying tissue laterally about 2.5 cm (1 inch) and hold it there securely				
Grasp the syringe with the last three fingers and inject the needle as for an intramuscular injection				
Test to see if the needle is in a vein by pulling back on the plunger with the forefinger and thumb				
If the needle is not in a vein, push the plunger in with the thumb				
Wait about 10 seconds after injecting the medication before withdrawing the needle				
Do not massage the area where the medication was given				
Subcutaneous Injection				
Observe techniques for giving an intramuscular injection with the following two exceptions:				
Select an appropriate site where subcutaneous tissue is abundant				
Hold the skin taut over injection site or grasp tissue, depending on the patient's condition and needle length				

C. This section allows you to examine your techniques for administering an intradermal injection.

Recommended Technique	S	N.I.	U	Comments
Select proper equipment and supplies and fill syringe with the proper agent				
Select an area on the inner aspect of the forearm properly				
Cleanse the intended site of entry with a pledget moistened with an antiseptic				

(continued)

Recommended Technique	S	N.I.	U	Comments
Hold the patient's arm in the hand and stretch the skin tautly with the thumb				
Place the needle almost flat against the skin, bevel side up				
Inject the needle about 1/16 inch and test whether the needle is in a vein				
Slowly inject the agent while watching for a small wheal or blister				
After injecting the agent slowly, withdraw the needle quickly				
Do not massage the area where the injection was made				
Observe the area for signs of a reaction at ordered intervals				

CHAPTER 35

Intravenous Medications

SUMMARY

Administering intravenous solutions, discussed in Chapter 15, can be considered a form of intravenous medication administration. It is used for fluid balance and maintenance. However, the focus of this chapter is on the methods for administering intravenous drugs and the techniques for using various venous-access devices, and not fluid therapy. The intravenous route includes peripheral and central veins.

MATCHING QUESTIONS

Directions: For items 1 through 5, match the terms in Part B with the descriptions in Part A.

Part A

1. _____ Used to administer undiluted medication quickly into a vein.
2. _____ Used to administer a parenteral drug that is diluted in 50 cc of solution over 30 to 60 minutes.
3. _____ Used to administer IV medication without circulatory overload.
4. _____ Used to administer parenteral medication in a large volume of blood.
5. _____ Used to provide the greatest protection against infection when IV medications are required frequently over a very long period of time.

Part B

a. Implanted catheter
b. Secondary infusion
c. Volume control set
d. Central venous catheter
e. Bolus

MULTIPLE CHOICE QUESTIONS

Directions: For items 1 through 10, circle the letter that corresponds to the best answer for each question.

1. Intravenous medications are usually added to a large volume of solution by the:
   a. Physician
   b. Pharmacist
   c. Manufacturer
   d. Nurse

2. Patients receiving medication via a central venous catheter over an extended period of time are most likely to have which of the following type of catheter:
   a. A percutaneous catheter
   b. An angio-catheter
   c. A tunneled catheter
   d. An implanted catheter

3. Goggles and respirator mask are recommended when preparing which of the following medications for administration:
   a. Anticoagulant drugs
   b. Parenteral drugs.
   c. Intravenous drugs
   d. Antineoplastic drugs

4. A Hickman catheter is an example of:
   a. A percutaneous, catheter
   b. An angio-catheter
   c. A tunneled catheter
   d. An implanted catheter

5. An intermittent infusion is one in which IV medication is given:
   a. Over an extended period of time
   b. All at one time
   c. Over a short period of time
   d. At a rate of 1 ml per minute

6. Bolus administration of intravenous medication has the greatest potential for:
   a. Causing life-threatening reactions
   b. Delivering the drug gradually
   c. Backfilling the tubing
   d. Allowing IV fluid to flow slowly

7. The best feature of a medication lock is that it:
   a. Facilitates the administration of medication
   b. Prevents medication errors
   c. Is a venous-access device
   d. Eliminates administration of unneeded IV fluids

8. A secondary infusion involves administering an IV medication that has been diluted in a volume of solution equal to:
   a. 500 to 1000 cc
   b. 250 to 500 cc
   c. 100 to 200 cc
   d. 50 to 100 cc

9. When caring for patients who are at risk for circulatory overload, it would be appropriate to administer IV medications using a:
   a. Volume-control set
   b. Central venous catheter
   c. Continuous infusion set
   d. Bolus administration

10. An advantage resulting from the use of multilumen central venous catheters is:
   a. Unused lumen can be capped with a medication lock
   b. They can be used for short-term intravenous therapy
   c. Incompatible substances can be given simultaneously
   d. They facilitate clearing the catheter of heparin

TRUE OR FALSE QUESTIONS

Directions: For items 1 through 10, decide if the statement is true or false and mark T or F in the space provided.

1. _____ Bolus is the term used to designate multiple-dose intravenous medications.

2. _____ A heparin lock is used for continuous intravenous medications.

3. _____ Implanted central venous catheters provide the greatest protection against infection.

4. _____ Antineoplastic drugs can be absorbed accidentally by health care professionals.

5. _____ Implanted ports can sustain about 2,000 punctures over several years.

6. _____ Tunneled catheters are inserted through the skin in a peripheral vein, such as the jugular.

7. _____ Older adults are more likely to experience adverse drug effects because there is more circulating protein-bound drug in the blood.

8. _____ The cost for administering intravenous drugs during home care is reimbursed by Medicare.

9. _____ A piggyback solution is a small volume of diluted medication that is connected to and positioned higher than the primary solution.

10. _____ A central venous catheter is a venous-access device that extends to the vena cava.

SHORT ANSWER QUESTIONS

Directions: Read each of the following statements and supply the word(s) necessary in the space provided.

1. List four steps (SASH) the nurse should follow when giving medication through a heparin lock.
   a. S =
   b. A =
   c. S =
   d. H =

2. List advantages given in this chapter for using a central venous catheter over a peripheral one.
   _____
   _____
   _____
   _____

3. List four reasons the intravenous route may be the preferred route of medication administration.

CRITICAL THINKING EXERCISE

This chapter includes recommendations for avoiding self-contamination when antineoplastic drugs are administered. Discuss how you would explain these precautions:
   a. When the patient is a young child _____
   _____
   _____
   b. When the patient is a teen _____
   _____
   _____

PERFORMANCE CHECKLIST

A. This section allows you to examine your technique for IV medication by continuous infusion.

1. Place a check mark in the "S" ("satisfactory") column if you used the recommended technique.
2. Place a check mark in the "N.I." ("needs improvement") column if you used some but not all of each recommended technique.

3. Place a check mark in the "U" ("unsatisfactory") column if you forgot to include that particular recommended technique.
4. The section for comment allows space to make notes about when further practice is indicated, what errors you made, suggestions that will improve your skills, and so on.

Recommended Technique	S	N.I.	U	Comments
Compare the MAR with the written medical order				
Observe for documented drug or food allergies				
Inspect current infusion site for swelling, redness, or tenderness				
Wash your hands				
Identify the patient				
Clamp the current infusion				
Swab the port on the container				
Instill the medication into the container				
Lower the container and gently rotate it to mix drug and solution				
Suspend solution and release clamp				
Regulate flow rate				
Attach a label to the container indicating the drug, dose, time, and your initials				
Record the medication on the MAR				
Observe the patient and the progress of the infusion at least hourly				
Record appropriate data on the required forms for documentation				

(continued)

B. This section allows you to examine your technique for administering an intermittent secondary infusion.

Recommended Technique	S	N.I.	U	Comments
Compare the MAR with the written medical order				
Observe the documented drug or food allergies				
Inspect current infusion site for swelling, redness, or tenderness				
Review drug action and side effects				
Remove refrigerated solution at least 30 minutes prior to use				
Check the drop factor on the package of secondary tubing; calculate the rate of infusion; have another nurse check your calculations				
Locate and swab the port; insert and tape the needle within the port				
Release the clamp on the secondary solution; regulate the rate of flow				
Clamp the tubing when the solution has instilled				
Rehang the primary container and readjust the flow rate				
Leave the secondary tubing in place if another secondary infusion is scheduled within 24 to 72 hours				
Record the appropriate data on the required forms for documentation				

C. This section allows you to examine your technique for using a volume-control set.

Recommended Technique	S	N.I.	U	Comments
Compare the MAR with the written medical order				
Observe for documented food and drug allergies				
Review drug action and side effects				
Assess the patient's fluid status				
Inspect current infusion site for redness, swelling, or tenderness				

Recommended Technique	S	N.I.	U	Comments
Determine the drop factor on the volume-control set; calculate the rate of infusion; have another nurse check your calculations				
Wash your hands and put on gloves				
Close all clamps on the volume-control set; insert spike into IV solution				
Seal air vent if the IV solution is in a plastic bag; leave it open if the container is glass				
Release the clamp above the fluid chamber				
Fill the calibrated chamber with about 30 cc of IV solution and tighten clamp				
Squeeze and release the drip chamber until it is one-half full				
Open lower clamp until the tubing is filled with fluid; reclamp				
Open clamp above the calibrated container; fill with desired volume				
Swab the injection port on the calibrated container				
Instill the prepared medication				
Rotate fluid chamber to mix				
Connect the tubing to the patient's IV catheter; release the lower clamp; regulate the drip				
Label the fluid chamber with drug, dose, time, and your initials				
Return before the medication is due to finish				
Release upper clamp when the medication is finished				
Refill the fluid chamber with the next hour's worth of fluid; readjust rate				
Remove the drug label				
Record the appropriate data on the required forms for documentation				

CHAPTER 36

Airway Management

SUMMARY

The primary function of the respiratory system is to facilitate ventilation so that there is appropriate exchange of oxygen and carbon dioxide at the cellular level. Adequate ventilation is dependent on clear air passages from the nose to the alveoli. This chapter presents information on various skills for promoting and assisting pulmonary function, including caring for the patient with an oral airway or a tracheostomy and removing secretions from the respiratory tract.

MATCHING QUESTIONS

Directions: For items 1 through 5, match the terms in Part B with the description in Part A.

Part A
1. _____ A type of secretion found in the respiratory tract.
2. _____ A secretion raised to the level of the upper airway
3. _____ A surgically created opening into the trachea
4. _____ Technique to loosen retained secretions
5. _____ A collective system of tubes found in the respiratory tract

Part B
a. Sputum
b. Tracheostomy
c. Airway
d. Vibration
e. Mucus

MULTIPLE CHOICE QUESTIONS

Directions: For items 1 through 12, circle the letter that corresponds to the best answer for each question.

1. To avoid narrowing of respiratory passageways and decreased volume of exchanged gases for patients with lung congestion, the nurse should:
   a. Encourage the patient to cough
   b. Encourage the patient to exercise
   c. Encourage adequate fluid intake
   d. Encourage adequate nutrition

2. The process of suspending droplets of water in a gas is known as:
   a. Humidification
   b. Atomization
   c. Nebulization
   d. Aerosolization

3. Postural drainage should be performed:
   a. Before breakfast and at bedtime
   b. Before meals and before bedtime
   c. After meals, three times a day
   d. At midmorning and mid-afternoon

4. The technique used when performing percussion is:
   a. Striking the chest with rhythmic gentle blows using a cupped hand
   b. Striking the chest with rhythmic gentle blows using open hands
   c. Using firm, strong, circular movements on the chest with open hands
   d. Using firm, strong, circular movements on the chest with cupped hands

5. The primary purpose for using percussion and vibration over an area of a lung is to:
   a. Move residual air out of the lung
   b. Force the patient to take deep breaths
   c. Cause thick secretions to break loose
   d. Prevent the air sacs in the lung from collapsing

235

6. The points of measurement for determining the appropriate size of oral airway to use are:
   a. The front is parallel with the front teeth and the back reaches the angle of the jaw
   b. The front is parallel with the front teeth and the back reaches the back of the throat
   c. The front is parallel with the tip of the nose and the back reaches the earlobe
   d. The front is parallel with the tip of the chin and the back reaches the earlobe

7. The best time of the day to collect a sputum specimen is:
   a. After a meal
   b. Between meals
   c. Upon awakening
   d. At bedtime

8. An oral airway should be briefly removed every:
   a. 1 hour
   b. 2 hours
   c. 3 hours
   d. 4 hours

9. Most agencies specify that the inner cannula of a tracheostomy should be cleaned at least every:
   a. 4 hours
   b. 8 hours
   c. 12 hours
   d. 24 hours

10. The catheter for suctioning a tracheostomy on an adult should be inserted no more than:
    a. 10–12.5 centimeter
    b. 15–20.5 centimeter
    c. 20–25.5 centimeter
    d. 25–30.5 centimeter

11. Patients are most likely to react to the sensation of suffocation with feelings of:
    a. Depression
    b. Fear
    c. Hopelessness
    d. Anger

12. The airway is protected by the epiglottis, which:
    a. Seals the airway when swallowing
    b. Keeps the trachea from collapsing
    c. Traps particulate matter
    d. Beats debris upward in the airway so it can be expectorated

TRUE OR FALSE QUESTIONS

Directions: For items 1 through 9, decide if the statement is true or false and mark T or F in the space provided.

1. _____ Postural drainage should be done before meals and at bedtime.

2. _____ Usually a pressure of 100 to 140 mm Hg is recommended when using a portable machine for suctioning a patient's airway.

3. _____ Suctioning should never be done routinely.

4. _____ A good time to collect a sputum specimen is following respiratory therapy treatments.

5. _____ The principles of medical asepsis must be followed when suctioning secretions from a tracheostomy.

6. _____ To ensure a sufficient quantity of specimen for study, it is best to collect at least 10 ml of sputum.

7. _____ Most adults can accommodate an 80-mm oral airway.

8. _____ If an airway is too long it will depress the epiglottis, thus potentiating the risk of airway obstruction.

9. _____ Because the tracheostomy tube is below the larynx, patients are able to talk.

SHORT ANSWER QUESTIONS

Directions: Read each of the following statements and supply the word(s) necessary in the space provided.

1. List the steps to follow when inserting an oral airway:
   _____
   _____
   _____
   _____
   _____

2. Identify the approaches for airway suctioning described in this chapter.
   _____
   _____
   _____
   _____

CRITICAL THINKING EXERCISES

1. Develop a plan for teaching a tracheostomy patient how to suction herself.
2. Determine assessment criteria that would indicate the need for suctioning:
   a. When the patient is an infant

   _____

   _____

   _____

   b. When the patient is an older adult

   _____

   _____

   _____

3. What essential points would you include when explaining how to collect a sputum specimen to a child?

PERFROMANCE CHECKLIST

A. This section allows you to examine your techniques for using postural drainage.
1. Place a check mark in the "S" ("satisfactory") column if you used the recommended technique.
2. Place a check mark in the "N.I." ("needs improvement") column if you used some but not all of each recommended technique.

3. Place a check mark in the "U" ("unsatisfactory") column if you forgot to include that particular recommended technique.
4. The section for comment allows space to make notes about when further practice is indicated, what errors you made, suggestions that will improve your skills, and so on.

Recommended Technique	S	N.I.	U	Comments
Use postural drainage before meals and at bedtime				
Administer prescribed medications that dilate respiratory passages before therapy				
Be familiar with positions the patient cannot safely assume				
Have tissues available for the patient for expectorating and coughing				
Know areas of the lungs to be drained and position the patient accordingly				
Allow the patient to assume positions for 15 to 30 minutes; 45 minutes if he can tolerate it				
Encourage the patient to cough and expectorate after each position				

B. This section allows you to examine your techniques for caring for a patient with a tracheostomy.

Recommended Technique	S	N.I.	U	Comments
Note the patient's respirations regularly for evidence of accumulations of mucus in the respiratory tract				
Encourage and help the patient raise secretions through the tracheostomy and wipe mucus away with lint-free material				

(continued)

Recommended Technique	S	N.I.	U	Comments
Provide suctioning whenever necessary while using a sterile catheter lubricated with normal saline				
Oxygenate the patient before, during, and after suctioning as indicated and permitted				
Instill 4 to 5 ml of normal saline into the tracheostomy if mucus is tenacious				
Test the equipment for proper functioning before suctioning				
Lubricate the catheter with normal saline before suctioning				
Insert the catheter 25 to 30 centimeters (10 to 12 inches) with the suction off, then suction both bronchi with gentle suction				
Rotate the catheter gently and move it up the respiratory tract while suctioning				
Use just enough suction to remove secretions and suction for no longer than 10 to 15 seconds at one time				
Remove the catheter to allow the patient to raise secretions if he coughs during suctioning				
Note that the inner and outer cannula are in place and well secured with tape				
See to it that there is a set of sterile equipment on hand in case of an emergency				
Follow strict aseptic technique at all times Administer oral hygiene to the patient regularly				
Observe precautions when the patient is receiving oxygen through the tracheostomy				

C. This section allows you to examine your techniques for using additional methods for assisting pulmonary functioning.

Recommended Technique	S	N.I.	U	Comments
Aerosolize medications				
Provide intermittent positive pressure breathing				
Use percussion and vibration				

CHAPTER 37

Resuscitation

SUMMARY

Nurses are often the first respondents when patients experience cardiopulmonary emergencies. This chapter reviews the most recent guidelines from the Emergency Cardiac Care Committee and Subcommittees of the American Heart Association for performing basic life support techniques. Age-related differences for performing CPR are also discussed.

MULTIPLE CHOICE QUESTIONS

Directions: For items 1 through 10, circle the letter that corresponds to the best answer for each question.

1. Of the following, which artery is recommended for checking the pulse of an adult during CPR?
   a. The femoral artery
   b. The radial artery
   c. The carotid artery
   d. The brachial artery

2. Before starting cardiac compressions, it is particularly important to:
   a. Be sure that the victim is not breathing
   b. Be sure that the victim is pulseless
   c. Be sure that the victim's head is tilted back
   d. Be sure that the victim is unconscious

3. Rescue breathing for an adult should be carried out every:
   a. 1 to 1 1/2 seconds for 5 seconds
   b. 5 seconds for 5 seconds
   c. 5 seconds for 1 1/2 seconds
   d. 1 to 1 1/2 seconds for 1 to 1 1/2 seconds

4. When performing CPR on an adult, the ratio of breaths per compressions should be:
   a. 5 breaths to every 5 compressions
   b. 1 breath to every 5 compressions
   c. 1 breath to every 15 compressions
   d. 2 breaths to every 15 compressions

5. The depth of chest compressions for an adult receiving CPR should be:
   a. 1/2 to 1 inch
   b. 1 to 1 1/2 inches
   c. 1 1/2 to 2 inches
   d. 2 to 3 inches

6. A state in which the response pattern of decreased energy reserves results in an individual's inability to maintain breathing adequate to support life describes which of the following nursing diagnoses:
   a. Inability to sustain spontaneous ventilation
   b. Impaired gas exchange
   c. Ineffective airway clearance
   d. Impaired cardiopulmonary tissue perfussion

7. In order to relieve an airway obstruction for an unconscious victim, you would:
   a. Place your fist in the middle of the abdomen
   b. Place the heel of your hand in the midline above the navel
   c. Place the fists in the middle of the breastbone
   d. Grasp the person about the abdomen from behind; tilt the head

8. Which of the following would indicate that a complete airway obstruction is present:
   a. The victim is unconscious
   b. Hearing an audible, high-pitched sound on inspiration
   c. The victim is not able to speak or cough
   d. The victim grasps his throat with his hands

9. The method of choice for opening the airway is:
   a. The head tilt-chin lift technique
   b. The jaw-thrust technique
   c. The chest-thrust technique
   d. The, subdiaphragmatic-thrust technique

10. The recovery position is best described as:
    a. A prone position
    b. A side-lying position
    c. A semi-Fowlers position
    d. A Trendelenberg position

TRUE OR FALSE QUESTIONS

Directions: For items 1 through 10, decide if the statement is true or false and mark T or F in the space provided.

1. _____ It is recommended that the carotid artery be used to check for a pulse when performing CPR on an infant.

2. _____ When starting CPR on an infant, only one initial rescue breath should be given.

3. _____ The ratio of breaths to chest compressions is 2 breaths to 15 compressions.

4. _____ There is always the risk of fracturing ribs when performing CPR.

5. _____ It is not possible to identify, in advance, the type of resuscitation one will allow.

6. _____ Some older adults fear that if they specify that they do not want to be resuscitated, they will receive inferior treatment.

7. _____ Patients who take daily doses of aspirin are more likely to bleed internally when chest compressions are administered.

8. _____ To dislodge an object from an infant's airway, a series of chest thrusts followed by a series of back blows are delivered.

9. _____ Before beginning cardiopulmonary resuscitation, shake the victim and shout her name.

10. _____ The decision to cease performing CPR is made by the first respondent.

SHORT ANSWER QUESTIONS

Directions: Read each of the following statements and supply the word(s) necessary in the space provided.

1. Identify the signs that are typical when a victim is choking on a foreign object.
   a. _____
   b. _____
   c. _____
   d. _____
   e. _____
   f. _____

2. Define the ABCs of basic life support.
   a. A is for _____
   b. B is for _____
   c. C is for _____

3. Identify the five criteria for interrupting CPR as presented in this chapter.
   a. _____
   b. _____
   c. _____
   d. _____
   e. _____

CRITICAL THINKING EXERCISES

1. Describe the adjustments that you would make when promoting cardiopulmonary functioning:
   a. When the patient is an infant _____
   _____
   _____

   b. When the patient is a child _____
   _____
   _____

2. Differences in cpr among infants, children, and adults
Directions: Review the chart below and fill in the missing
information.

Technique	Infant (to 1 year)	Child (1 to 8 years)	Adult (8 years and older)
Rescue Breaths:			
Initial:	2 breaths	2 breaths	2 breaths
Subsequent breaths:	1 every 3 seconds	1 every _____	1 every 5 seconds
Rate:	_____	20/minute	_____
Duration:	1 to 1½ seconds	1 to 1½ seconds	1 to 1½ seconds
Compressions:			
Location:	In the midline, one finger's width below the nipples	_____ _____ _____	Two finger widths above the tip of the sternum
Hand use:	Two or three fingers	Heel of one hand	Two hands
Rate:	At least 100/minute	_____	80–100/minute
Depth:	_____	1 to 1½ seconds	1 to 1½ seconds or more

PERFORMANCE CHECKLIST

A. This section allows you to examine your techniques for providing measures to relieve choking.

1. Place a check mark in the "S" ("satisfactory") column if you used the recommended technique.
2. Place a check mark in the "N.I." ("needs improvement") column if you used some but not all of each recommended technique.

3. Place a check mark in the "U" ("unsatisfactory") column if you forgot to include that particular recommended technique.
4. The section for comment allows space to make notes about when further practice is indicated, what errors you made, suggestions that will improve your skills, and so on.

Recommended Technique	S	N.I.	U	Comments
Encourage coughing if the choking victim can talk				
If coughing cannot be done to dislodge a foreign object, then:				
Stand behind the victim and allow him to lean over your arm with his head lower than his chest				
Stand behind the victim and place your arms around the victim's abdomen				
Make a fist with one hand and grab it with the other hand				
Place the fist against the victim's abdomen, slightly below the rib cage and above the navel				
Allow the victim to fall forward over your arms				
Press the fist into the victim's abdomen with a forceful upward thrust				
Repeat the maneuver if necessary 6 to 10 times				
If unsuccessful, begin cardiopulmonary resuscitation as indicated by the patient's condition				

(continued)

B. This section allows you to examine your techniques for administering cardiopulmonary resuscitation to an adult.

Recommended Technique	S	N.I.	U	Comments
Place the victim on a firm surface, such as the floor or a bedboard				
Place one rescuer alongside patient's head, the other on the opposite side near the patient's chest				
Before starting rescue breathing, tilt victim's head backward, lift at the neck, and press down the forehead or Thrust the victim's jaw forward to open the airway if the above maneuver does not work				
Take a deep breath, pinch the victim's nostrils shut, and forcefully blow your breath into the victim's open mouth				
Repeat the above rescue breathing for a total of four times quickly				
After the initial four, give one rescue breath every 5 seconds after five cardiac compressions				
To give cardiac compressions, place the heel of one hand over the long axis of the lower half of the sternum				
Place the second hand over the first and interlock your fingers; keep hands about 3.75 centimeters (1 1/2 inches) above xiphoid process				
Exert pressure on the sternum by bringing the shoulders over the hands and keep the elbows and arms straight				
Depress the sternum about 3.75 to 5 centimeters (1 1/2 to 2 inches) with each compression and then release pressure immediately				
Continue with compressions at the rate of 80 per minute and keep hands properly positioned over the victim always				
Check effectiveness of CPR by noting skin color, and pulse				
Continue with CPR as long as the victim's heart does not beat spontaneously				
Adjust the above techniques correctly when there is only one rescuer				

C. This section allows you to examine your techniques for using a self-inflating bag and mask.

Recommended Technique	S	N.I.	U	Comments
Stand or kneel at the victim's head				
Place the mask firmly over the victim's nose and mouth and hold his chin up and back to open the airway				
Squeeze the bag to force inhalation and quickly release pressure for exhalation				
Compress the bag at the average normal respiratory rate unless the victim's condition indicates otherwise				

CHAPTER 38

Death and Dying

SUMMARY

This chapter provides information on many aspects of the dying and grieving experiences. The unique emotional, spiritual, and physical problems of the terminally ill are discussed.

The purposes of this chapter is to assist students with exploring their own attitudes and feelings about death and to identify the nurse's role in helping terminally ill patients die with dignity. The concepts of grief and loss are also explored.

MATCHING QUESTIONS

Directions: For items 1 through 5, match the typical emotional responses in Part B with the stages according to Kübler-Ross in Part A.

Part A

1. _____ First stage
2. _____ Second stage
3. _____ Third stage
4. _____ Fourth stage
5. _____ Fifth stage

Part B

a. Bargaining
b. Acceptance
c. Denial and isolation
d. Depression
e. Anger

MULTIPLE CHOICE QUESTIONS

Directions: For items 1 through 10, circle the letter that corresponds to the best answer for each question.

1. An advanced directive is:
   a. A statement of the dying person's funeral arrangements
   b. A statement giving the family the right to make final decisions
   c. A statement describing the person's wishes about his care when death is near
   d. A statement describing the person's wishes about his estate when death is near

2. The third stage of dying according to Kübler-Ross is:
   a. Denial
   b. Anger
   c. Bargaining
   d. Acceptance

3. Anger, according to Kübler-Ross, is considered to be the:
   a. First stage
   b. Second stage
   c. Fourth stage
   d. Fifth stage

4. When the family is physically and emotionally unable to care for the dying member in the home, care must be taken to:
   a. Arrange for financial coverage for the patient
   b. Arrange for a special agency for the dying
   c. See that the family is not made to feel guilty
   d. See that the family understands the hospital routine

5. The emphasis of hospice care is:
   a. Helping the patient live until he dies
   b. Helping the patient with his hygiene needs
   c. Teaching the family members to care for the patient
   d. Providing counseling for the patient and family

6. The nurse can facilitate moving to the stage of acceptance wherein the patient can die in peace and dignity by:
   a. Responding to emotional needs
   b. Sustaining realistic hope
   c. Accepting reality
   d. Understanding common fears

7. Of the following, which is considered the last reflex to disappear as death approaches:
   a. Sucking
   b. Gagging
   c. Blinking
   d. Swallowing

8. Of the following pain-relief measures, which would give the dying patient the best relief:
   a. Teaching her techniques such as imagery and relaxation
   b. Administering medication only when it is absolutely necessary
   c. Administering the pain medication on a routine schedule
   d. Explaining that most pain medications may cause addiction

9. Which of the following signs is the one that is most positive that death has occurred:
   a. The absence of heartbeats
   b. The absence of respirations
   c. The absence of blood pressure
   d. The absence of brain waves

10. A coroner has the right to order an autopsy to be performed if:
    a. The physician requests it
    b. The patient was a child
    c. The death was of a suspicious nature
    d. The death happened in the hospital

TRUE OR FALSE QUESTIONS

Directions: For items 1 through 12, decide if the statement is true or false and mark T or F in the space provided.

1. _____ Denial is an avoidance technique used to separate oneself from situations that are threatening or unpleasant.

2. _____ It is important to understand one's personal feelings about death and dying before providing terminal care.

3. _____ Even though an individual donates his organs, in many states the next of kin must sign a permit before the organs are removed from the body.

4. _____ According to Dr. Elisabeth Kübler-Ross, all people go through the five stages of dying in the same order.

5. _____ Each of the five stages of dying last for a specified time and they are sequential.

6. _____ Even though an individual is considered competent, the physician may not allow him to refuse treatment.

7. _____ Sometimes individuals may prolong dying while awaiting a sign that others are prepared to accept the loss.

8. _____ As death approaches, the patient's temperature lowers and her skin becomes cold and clammy.

9. _____ Pain can be intensified by fear and anxiety.

10. _____ The death rattle is caused by the patient's inability to expectorate sputum.

11. _____ When death is imminent, the patient's pain often increases.

12. _____ The physician's signature is required on the death certificate only when the cause of death is suspicious.

SHORT ANSWER QUESTIONS

Directions: Read each of the following statements and supply the word(s) necessary in the space provided.

1. Identify six signs suggested in this chapter that usually clearly indicate that death is imminent.
   a. _____
   b. _____
   c. _____
   d. _____
   e. _____
   f. _____

2. Identify seven suggestions for summoning the family of a dying person.

   a. _____

   b. _____

   c. _____

   d. _____

   e. _____

   f. _____

   g. _____

3. Identify five common physical reactions grieving individuals may experience.

   a. _____

   b. _____

   c. _____

   d. _____

   e. _____

4. List four examples of pathologic grief.

   a. _____

   b. _____

   c. _____

   d. _____

CRITICAL THINKING EXERCISE

Describe adjustments you make when caring for the terminally ill:

   a. When the patient is an infant or child _____
   _____

   b. When the patient is elderly _____
   _____

PERFORMANCE CHECKLIST

A. This section allows you to examine your techniques for offering support to someone who is terminally ill.

1. Place a check mark in the "S" ("satisfactory") column if you used the recommended technique.
2. Place a check mark in the "N.I." ("needs improvement") column if you used some but not all of each recommended technique.
3. Place a check mark in the "U" ("unsatisfactory") column if you forgot to include that particular recommended technique.
4. The section for comment allows space to make notes about when further practice is indicated, what errors you made, suggestions that will improve your skills, and so on.

Recommended Technique	S	N.I.	U	Comments
Take steps to examine your own feelings about life, death, and dying				
Show understanding for the patient's feelings and for those of her family				
Provide a nonjudgmental atmosphere and listen to the patient and her family				
Show an understanding of how attitudes toward death differ among people				
Observe for fear of death and offer appropriate support				
Support hope, even when the prognosis is poor, in an appropriate manner				
Show an understanding of what to tell the patient and her family about terminal illness				
Respect a rational adult's right to refuse further therapy				
Assist appropriately to meet a patient's spiritual needs during a terminal illness				

(continued)

B. This section allows you to examine your techniques for offering personal care to a patient who is terminally ill.

Recommended Technique	S	N.I.	U	Comments
Facet of Care				
Nutrition				
Intestinal and urinary elimination				
Mouth, nose, and eye care				
Care of the skin and mucous membranes				
Positioning in bed				
Environmental considerations				
Provision for the proper relief of pain				

C. This section allows you to examine your techniques for assisting the family of the patient who is terminally ill.

Recommended Technique	S	N.I.	U	Comments
Strive to meet the various needs of family members when a patient is terminally ill				
Allow family members to help with the care of the patient when appropriate				
Use appropriate measures when relatives are critical of care				
Offer appropriate emotional support when the patient dies				
Show an understanding of the grieving process				

D. This section allows you to examine your techniques for performing postmortem care.

Recommended Technique	S	N.I.	U	Comments
Transfer any patient who shared a room with the deceased temporarily to another room				
Notify the nursing administration office and the health agency switchboard				
Contact any individuals involved in organ procurement. Inform the designated mortician that the patient has died				
Assemble all the equipment for cleaning, wrapping, and identifying the body				
Determine that the family and clergyman have spent all the time they want with the body				

Recommended Technique	S	N.I.	U	Comments
Place the body supine with the arms extended at the side or folded over the abdomen				
Remove hairpins and clips				
Close the eyelids by applying gentle pressure				
Replace or retain the dentures within the mouth				
Use a small towel under the chin to close an open mouth				
Leave all equipment in place if this is a suspected crime				
Remove all equipment if the patient died of natural causes				
Apply gloves and dispose of all contaminated and soiled articles				
Cleanse the soiled areas of the body				
Apply disposable pads to the perineal area				
Attach an identification tag either to the ankle or the wrist and leave the agency identification bracelet intact				
Remove or make an inventory of the valuables still attached to the body				
Wrap the body with a shroud				
Attach an identification tag to the shroud				
Transport the body to the morgue or wait for the arrival of the mortician				
Arrange for all valuables to be locked until claimed by the family				
Complete the patient's permanent record indicating in what manner the body was removed				

Correct Answers and Rationale

CHAPTER 1

Nursing Foundations

The number in parentheses following each rationale indicates on which page in *Fundamental Skills and Concepts in Patient Care,* Seventh Edition, you can find the correct answer.

ANSWERS TO MATCHING QUESTIONS

Items 1 Through 4 (Refer to Table 12)

1. (c)
2. (a)
3. (d)
4. (b)

Items 5 Through 8 (Refer to Page 17)

5. (d) Assessment skills are those skills used by the nurse for observing, interviewing, and examining a patient.
6. (c) Caring skills are those skills that restore or maintain an individual's health.
7. (a) The nurse uses comforting skills to convey security and stability during crisis.
8. (b) Nurses use counseling skills for communication that involves both talking and active listening.

Items 9 Through 16

9. (e) An art is the ability to perform an act skillfully. (8)
10. (i) Active listening is demonstrating full attention to what is being said and hearing the content being communicated, as well as the unspoken message. (17)
11. (d) Caring is the concern and attachment that occurs from the close relationship of one human being with another. (17)
12. (a) Empathy is an intuitive awareness of what the patient is experiencing. This skill involves being able to remain compassionate yet detached. (17)

13. (f) Nursing is the diagnosis and treatment of human responses to actual or potential health problems (ANA, 1980). (9)
14. (c) A theory is an opinion, belief, or view that explains a process. (9)
15. (h) A science is a body of knowledge unique to a particular subject. (9)
16. (j) Sympathy is feeling so similarly to the patient that the nurse becomes ineffective in providing for the patient's needs. (17)

ANSWERS TO TRUE OR FALSE QUESTIONS

Items I Through 6

1. *True.*
2. *False.* In the midst of deplorable health care conditions, Florence Nightingale, an Englishwoman born of wealthy parents, announced that she, had been called by God to become a nurse.
3. *True.*
4. *True.*
5. *False.* It may be expected that as the role of the nurse changes in the future, there will be further revisions to the definition of nursing in order to describe more succinctly the scope of nursing practice. (9)
6. *False.* The nurse provides pertinent health information without offering specific advice. (17)

ANSWERS TO MULTIPLE CHOICE QUESTIONS

Items 1 Through 12

1. (c) The service of caring for the sick changed with the schism between King Henry VIII of England and the Catholic Church when nuns and priests were extradited to continental Europe. (5, 6)

259

2. (a)   Servicemen and their families alike were grateful; the country adored her. To show their appreciation, funds were donated to sustain the great work Florence Nightingale had begun.   (7)

3. (b)   In her writing and speaking, Henderson proposed that nursing is more than carrying out medical orders. It involves a special relationship and service between the nurse and those entrusted to his or her care.

4. (d)   Mildred Montag, a doctoral student, hypothesized that nursing education could be shortened to two years and relocated to a vocational school or a junior or community college. The graduate from this type of program would acquire an associate degree in nursing.   (12)

5. (a)   See Table 12.   (10)

6. (c)   See Table 12.   (10)

7. Before the nurse can determine what nursing care a person requires, the patient's needs and problems must be determined. This requires the use of assessment skills. The patient and family are the primary sources for information.   (17)

8. (d)   The unique function of the nurse is to assist the individual, sick or well, in the performance of those activities contributing to health or its recovery (or to a peaceful death) that he could perform unaided if he had the necessary strength, will or knowledge and to do it in such a way as to help him gain independence as rapidly as possible.   (17)

9. (b)   A counselor is one who listens to a client's needs, responds with information based upon his or her area of expertise, and facilitates the outcome a client desires. Once the patient's perspective is clear, the nurse provides pertinent health information without offering specific advice. Nurses promote the right of all individuals to make their own decisions and choices on matters affecting health and illness care. The role of the nurse is to share information on potential alternatives, allow patients the freedom to choose, and support the decision that is made.   (17)

10. (a)   A science is a body of knowledge unique to a particular subject. It develops from observing and studying the relation of one phenomenon to another. By developing a unique body of scientific knowledge, it is now possible to predict which nursing interventions are most appropriate for producing desired outcomes.   (9)

11. (b)   The most recent definition of nursing comes from the American Nurses' Association.   (9)

12. (d)   Continuing education is any planned learning experience that takes place beyond one's basic nursing program (ANA, 1974).   (13)

ANSWERS TO SHORT ANSWER QUESTIONS

1. Criteria used to select applicants include (refer to Page 7):
   a. Between the ages of 35 and 50
   b. Matronly and plainlooking
   c. Educated
   d. Serious disposition, neat, orderly, sober, industrious
   e. Must submit two letters of recommendation attesting to their moral character, integrity, and capacity to care for the sick

2. (Refer to Display 12)   (13)

3. Factors affecting the choice of nursing education programs include (refer to pages 9 and 11):
   a. A person's career goals
   b. Geographic location of schools
   c. Costs, involved
   d. Length of programs
   e. Reputation and success of past graduates
   f. Flexibility in course scheduling
   g. Opportunity for parttime versus fulltime enrollment
   h. Ease of articulation into the next level of education

4. Factors delaying the decision include (refer to Page 12):
   a. The date for implementation coincided with a national shortage of nurses.
   b. There was tremendous opposition from non-degree nurses who felt threatened that their titles and positions would be jeopardized.
   c. Employers of nurses feared that paying higher salaries to degreed personnel would escalate budgets beyond their financial limits.

5. (Refer to Table 13)   (12)

	Practical/Vocational Nurse	**Associate Degree Nurse**	**Baccalaureate Nurse**
Assess:	Gathers data from person with common health problems with predictable outcomes	Collects data from persons with complex health problems with unpredictable outcomes	Identifies data required to provide an appropriate nursing database
Diagnosis:	Contributes to the development of nursing diagnoses	Uses a classification list to write a nursing diagnostic statement	Conducts clinical tests of approved nursing diagnoses
Plan:	Assists in developing a written plan of care	Develops a written, individualized plan of care with specific nursing orders that reflects the standards for nursing practice	Plans care for healthy or sick individuals or groups in structured health care agencies or the community
Implement:	Performs basic nursing care under the direction of a registered nurse	Identifies priorities; directs others to carry out nursing orders	Applies nursing theory to the approaches used for resolving health problems of individuals or groups
Evaluate:	Contributes to the revision of the plan of care	Makes revisions in the plan of care	Conducts research that may improve nursing care

CHAPTER 2

Nursing Process

The number in parentheses following each rationale indicates on which page in *Fundamental Skills and Concepts in Patient Care,* Seventh Edition, you can find the correct answer.

ANSWERS TO MATCHING QUESTIONS

Items 1 Through 5

1. c (21)
2. e (25)
3. a (26)
4. d (28)
5. b (30)

Items 6 Through 11

6. b
7. b
8. a
9. a
10. b
11. a

ANSWERS TO MULTIPLE CHOICE QUESTIONS

Items 1 Through 15

1. (c) In the distant past, nursing practice involved actions that were based mostly on common sense and the examples set by older, more experienced nurses. Now nurses are planning and implementing patient care more independently. Nurses are being held responsible and accountable for providing appropriate patient care that reflects current accepted standards for nursing practice. (21)

2. (b) The nursing process is goal directed. It facilitates a united effort between the patient and the nursing team in achieving desired outcomes. (21)

3. (b) Data is either objective or subjective. Objective data is information that is observable and measurable, such as the patient's blood pressure. Subjective data is information that only the patient feels and can describe, such as pain. (22)

4. (c) Diagnosis, the second step in the nursing process, involves identifying problems. (25)

5. (b) The nursing process is dynamic. Since the health status of any patient is constantly changing, the nursing process acts like a continuous loop. Evaluation, the last step in the nursing process, involves data collection and the process begins again. (22)

6. (a) A characteristic of the nursing process is that it is patient centered. The nursing process facilitates a comprehensive plan of care for each patient as a unique individual. (22)

7. (c) Assessment, the first step in the nursing process, is the systematic collection and organization of data. (22)

8. (b) Collaborative problems are certain physiologic complications that nurses monitor to detect onset or change in status. Because they are beyond the independent scope of nursing practice, their management requires the combined expertise of the nurse and the physician. (26)

9. (a) A nursing diagnostic statement includes three parts: the problem, the etiology, and the signs and symptoms. (25)

10. (b) A nursing diagnosis is a three-part statement. It contains the diagnostic category or problem, the cause of the problem or etiology, and the signs and symptoms that the patient with a particular diagnosis is experiencing. (See Display 2-4) (25)

11. (a)   Not all of the patient's problems may be resolved during a typically short hospitalization. Prioritization involves ranking problems from most to least importance. One method, which is frequently used by nurses, is to rank nursing diagnoses according to Maslow's Hierarchy of Human Needs.   (26)

12. (d)   This choice is the best example because the statement shows the expected outcome, or the desired end result, for which one works. Johnny will walk, unassisted, to the playroom by a specific date. The other choices are not as specific in their terminology or in the date on which they will be accomplished.   (26–27)

13. (a)   The best nursing order in this situation states how much fluid (2 ounces), what kind of fluid (clear), and how often (every 2 hours until 10 p.m.). The other choices are not as specific in their directions and therefore could be misinterpreted. (See Display 2-8)   (30)

14. (c)   Evaluation is the process of determining if, or how well, a goal has been reached. It helps to determine the effectiveness of the plan of care.   (30)

15. (d)   When evaluation results show that a goal has not been met, modifications and revisions in the nursing care may be necessary. (See Display 2-9, page 31)

ANSWERS TO TRUE OR FALSE QUESTIONS

Items 1 Through 10

1. *False.* The information may be gathered in different ways, such as by asking the patient or family questions, making observations while examining the patient, reading the patient's record, and asking other health workers about their observations of the patient.   (23)

2. *False.* A nursing diagnosis is a statement describing a health problem that has the possibility of being resolved completely through nursing measures.   (25)

3. *True.*

4. *False.* Nurses commonly prioritize problems in reference to the hierarchy; however, there may be other methods to do this effectively.   (26)

5. *True.*

6. *True.*

7. *False.* Evaluation is the process of measuring how well a goal is reached.   (30)

8. *True.*

9. *False.* Subjective data is information that only the patient can experience and describe.   (22)

10. *True.*

ANSWERS TO SHORT ANSWER QUESTION

Items 1 and 2 (Refer to Page 21)

1. The etiology is: immobility

2. The problem is: impaired skin integrity

CHAPTER 3

Laws and Ethics

The number in parentheses following each rationale indicates on which page in *Fundamental Skills and Concepts in Patient Care,* Seventh Edition, you can find the correct answer.

ANSWERS TO MATCHING QESTIONS

Items 1 Through 6

(Refer to pages 37–40)
(These words are either listed as Key Terms or bolded in the text.)

1. (d)   4. (h)
2. (b)   5. (a)
3. (f)   6. (c)

Items 7 Through 12

(Refer to pages 35–37)

7. (e)   10. (b)
8. (f)   11. (d)
9. (c)   12. (a)

ANSWERS TO MULTIPLE CHOICE QUESTIONS

Items 1 Through 10

1. (a) A tort is litigation in which one citizen asserts that an injury, which may be physical, emotional, or financial, occurred as a consequence of another citizen's actions or failure to act. (37)

2. (d) Many statements of patient rights have been established. One that is widely used and distributed has been prepared by the American Hospital Association. (See Display 3-5) (44)

3. (b) An incident report is a written account of an unusual event involving a client, employee, or visitor that has the potential for being injurious. (41)

4. (d) Unintentional torts involve situations that result in an injury, although the person responsible did not purposely mean to cause harm. Cases of unintentional torts involve allegations of negligence or malpractice. (40)

5. (c) Good Samaritan laws, a name based on the biblical story of the person who gave aid to a beaten stranger along a roadside, have been enacted in many states. These laws provide legal immunity for passersby who provide emergency first aid to accident victims. None of the Good Samaritan laws provide absolute exemption from prosecution in the event of injury. Nurses, and others, are held to a higher standard of care since they have training above and beyond that of average lay persons. (41)

6. (d) The word *ethics* comes from a Greek word that means customs or modes of conduct. Ethics refers to moral or philosophical principles that direct actions as being either right or wrong. Various groups, such as nurses, have identified standards for ethical practice. (41)

7. (d) A code of ethics is a list of written statements describing ideal behavior. (See Display 3-4) (41 & 43)

8. (a) A nurse practice act is a form of state legislation that legally defines the unique role of the nurse and differentiates it from other health care practitioners. (36)

9. (a) Each state's board of nursing is the regulatory agency for managing the provisions of its nurse practice acts. The board of nursing develops rules and regulations for the education and licensing of individuals who wish to practice as nurses within the state. (36)

10. (a) Deontology refers to ethical study based on duty or moral obligations, decisions must be based on the ultimate morality of the act itself. (43)

ANSWERS TO TRUE OR FALSE QUESTIONS

Items 1 Through 10

1. *True.*
2. *False.* False imprisonment is the unjustifiable restraint or prevention of the movement of a person without proper consent. (38)
3. *True.*
4. *True.*
5. *True.*
6. *False.* The physician is responsible for giving the patient information about his medical treatment.
7. *True.*
8. *True.*
9. *False.* The person accused of breaking the law is called the defendant. (37)
10. *True.*

ANSWERS TO SHORT ANSWER QUESTIONS

Items 1 and 2

1. Elements that must be proven include (See Display 3-2, page 40):
   a. Duty
   b. Breach of duty
   c. Causation
   d. Injury
2. Ethical issues that nurses encounter include (See page 46):
   a. Telling the truth
   b. Protecting the patient's confidentiality
   c. Ensuring that the patient's wishes regarding various treatments are followed
   d. Advocating for the nondiscriminatory allocation of scarce resources
   e. Reporting incompetent or unethical practices

C H A P T E R   4

Health and Illness

The number in parentheses following each rationale indicates on which page in *Fundamental Skills and Concepts in Patient Care,* Seventh Edition, you can find the correct answer.

ANSWERS TO MATCHING QUESTIONS

Items 1 Through 12

(Refer to Figure 4-3, page 49)

1.	(c)	7.	(a)
2.	(a)	8.	(c)
3.	(b)	9.	(a)
4.	(b)	10.	(a)
5.	(d)	11.	(a)
6.	(a)	12.	(a)

ANSWERS TO MULTIPLE CHOICE QUESTIONS

Items 1 Through 12

1. (c)   In the preamble of its constitution, the World Health Organization (WHO) defines health as a state of complete physical, mental, and social well-being and not merely the absence of disease or infirmity.   (47)
2. (a)   The term *morbidity* refers to the incidence of a specific disease, disorder, or injury. The morbidity rate refers to the number of people affected. Statistics may be compiled on the basis of age, gender, or per 1000 people within the population.   (49)
3. (d)   The state of wellness is a full and balanced integration of physical, emotional, social, and spiritual health. Physical health exists when body organs function normally. Emotional health results when one feels safe. Social health is an outcome of feeling accepted and useful. Spiritual health is a feeling that one's life has purpose.   (48)

4. (c)   An acute illness is one that comes on suddenly and lasts a relatively short time. Answer (a) describes chronic illness. Answer (b) describes terminal illness. Answer (d) describes primary illness.   (49)
5. (c)   An idiopathic illness is one for which there is no known explanation for its development. Treatment of idiopathic illness generally focuses on relieving the signs and symptoms of the disease.   (50)
6. (b)   One method for administering nursing care is the functional method. When this approach is used, each nurse on a patient unit is assigned specific tasks.   (52)
7. (b)   Providing nursing care by the case method involves assigning one nurse to administer all the care a patient needs for a designated period of time. The case method is most often used in home health and public health nursing.   (52)
8. (c)   In team nursing, many nursing personnel divide the patient care and all work until it is completed. The personnel are organized and directed by a nurse called the "team leader." The team leader usually supervises the team.   (53)
9. (b)   A new way of administering nursing care is called nurse-managed care or case management. It is similar to the principles practiced by a successful business.   (53)
10. (a)   The term *continuity of care* refers to a continuum of health care. The goal is to avoid causing a patient, whether healthy or ill, to feel isolated, fragmented, or abandoned during the transfer from one type of health care services to another.   (53)

ANSWERS TO TRUE OR FALSE QUESTIONS

Items 1 Through 10

1. *False.* A chronic illness is an illness that comes on slowly and lasts a relatively long time.   (49)
2. *False.* Functional nursing is the least-practiced method of giving nursing care in this country.   (52)

266

3. *False. Physical* health is a state in which body organs function normally. Health is a state of complete physical, mental, and social well-being. (48)
4. *True.*
5. *True.*
6. *False.* Spiritual well-being is characterized as feeling one's life is purposeful. (48)
7. *True.*
8. *True.*
9. *False.* A resource is a possession that is valuable because its supply is limited and it has no substitute. Therefore, health is considered a resource. (48)
10. *True.*

EXAMPLE OF AN ANSWER TO THE DISCUSSION QUESTION

Method of Administration	Characteristics	Individual Responsible	Advantage/ Disadvantage	Health Care Setting
Primary Nursing				
Team Nursing				
Functional Nursing				
Nurse-Managed Care				

CHAPTER 5

Homeostasis, Adaptation, and Stress

The number in parentheses following each rationale indicates on which page in *Fundamental Skills and Concepts in Patient Care,* Seventh Edition, you can find the correct answer.

ANSWERS TO MATCHING QUESTIONS

Items 1 Through 6

(Refer to pages 55–63)

1. (d)	4. (e)
2. (f)	5. (b)
3. (c)	6. (a)

Items 7 Through 12

(Refer to Table 5-1, page 56)

7. (d)	10. (d)
8. (c)	11. (b)
9. (a)	12. (c)

Items 13 Through 20

(Refer to Table 5-4, page 63)

13. (c)	17. (b)
14. (f)	18. (e)
15. (a)	19. (h)
16. (g)	20. (d)

ANSWERS TO MULTIPLE CHOICE QUESTIONS

Items 1 Through 8

1. (c)   Homeostasis is the term used to describe a relatively stable state of physiologic equilibrium or balance. It literally means "staying the same." Although it sounds contradictory, staying the same requires constant physiologic activity.   (55)

2. (b)   The autonomic nervous system, which is subdivided into the sympathetic and parasympathetic nervous system, is composed of peripheral nerves that affect physiologic functions that are largely automatic and beyond voluntary control.   (58)

3. (d)   The parasympathetic nervous system tends to restore equilibrium after the danger is no longer present. It does so by inhibiting the physiologic stimulation of the sympathetic nervous system. The sympathetic nervous system prepares the body for the "fight or flight" response.   (58)

4. (b)   Behaving in a manner that is characteristic of a younger age is the coping mechanism known as regression. (See Table 5-4)   (63)

5. (a)   The general adaptation syndrome (GAS) refers to the collective physiologic processes that take place in response to a stressor.   (60)

6. (d)   The Social Readjustment Rating Scale was developed by Holmes and Rahe (1967). It is used to predict a person's potential for developing a stress-related disorder.   (61)

7. (b)   Powerlessness is an example of a psychological stressor. (See Table 5-1)   (56)

8. (a)   Rapid heart rate, rapid breathing, and dry mouth are examples of physical signs and symptoms of stress. (See Table 5-3)   (60)

ANSWERS TO TRUE OR FALSE QUESTIONS

Items 1 Through 10

1. *True.*
2. *False.* Forgetfulness is a cognitive symptom of increased stress. (See Table 5-3)   (60)
3. *True.*
4. *False.* The general adaptation syndrome refers to the collective physiologic process that takes place in response to a stressor.   (60)
5. *True.*

6. *True.*
7. *False.* Irritability, withdrawal, and depression are common *emotional* signs and symptoms of stress. (See Table 5-3)   (60)
8. *True.*

9. *False.* Bruxism is a term that refers to "tooth grinding." (See Display 5-1, page 61)
10. *False.* Accusing a person of a race different from one's own of being prejudiced is an example of projection. (See Table 5-4)   (63)

CHAPTER 6

Culture and Ethnicity

The number in parentheses following each rationale indicates on which page in *Fundamental Skills and Concepts in Patient Care*, Seventh Edition, you can find the correct answer.

ANSWERS TO MATCHING QUESTIONS

Items 1 Through 5

(These are Key Terms; refer to text pages 67–69)

1. (b)
2. (d)
3. (e)
4. (c)
5. (a)

Items 6 Through 10

(Refer to Table 6-5, page 76)

6. (c)
7. (e)
8. (a)
9. (d)
10. (b)

ANSWERS TO MULTIPLE CHOICE QUESTIONS

Items 1 Through 9

1. (b)   Transcultural nursing, a term coined by Madeline Leininger in the 1970s, refers to providing nursing care within the context of another's culture. Culturally sensitive care requires planning care within the patient's health belief system to achieve the best health outcome.   (70)

2. (a)   Currently, there are approximately 270 Indian tribes in the United States, with the Navajos being the largest surviving group.   (72)
3. (b)   See Table 6-3.   (75)
4. (c)   See Table 6-3.   (75)
5. (a)   Lactase is a digestive enzyme that converts lactose, the sugar in milk, into the simpler sugars glucose and galactose. A lactase deficiency causes an intolerance to dairy products.   (73)
6. (d)   All choices are correct.   (65)
7. (c)   See Table 6-4.   (75)
8. (a)   See Table 6-5.   (76)
9. (d)   The health practices that are unique to a particular group of individuals are sometimes referred to as "folk medicine." Folk medicine has come to mean those methods of disease prevention or treatment that are outside the mainstream of conventional practices. Folk medicine is often provided by lay rather than formally educated and licensed individuals.   (75)

ANSWERS TO TRUE OR FALSE QUESTIONS

Items 1 Through 10

1. *False.* It is wrong to assume that all individuals who affiliate with a particular group behave exactly alike. This is an example of stereotyping.   (70)
2. *True.*
3. *True.*
4. *True.*
5. *True.*
6. *False.* When it is possible to choose from several translators, select one who is the same gender as the patient and approximately the same age. Some patients may feel embarrassed to relate personal information to someone with whom they have little in common.   (71)

7. *False.* If the patient speaks some English, speak slowly, using simple words and short sentences. Lengthy or complex sentences are barriers to communicating with someone who is not skilled in English. If the patient appears confused by a question, repeat it slowly, without changing the words. Rephrasing tends to compound the patient's confusion as it forces him or her to translate yet another group of unfamiliar words.   (71)
8. *True.*
9. *False.* Prayer and penance, spiritual healers, and eating foods that are "hot" or "cold" are common health practices among Latinos.   (76)
10. *True.*

ANSWERS TO SHORT ANSWER QUESTIONS

Items 1 and 2

1. You may choose any five of the examples cited in Display 6-1.   (69)
2. You may choose any of the examples cited on pages 75–76 under the topic "Culturally Sensitive Nursing."

CHAPTER 7

The Nurse-Patient Relationship

The number in parentheses following each rationale indicates on which page in *Fundamental Skills and Concepts in Patient Care,* Seventh Edition, you can find the correct answer.

ANSWERS TO MATCHING QUESTIONS

Items 1 Through 6

(Refer to Table 7-1, page 84)

1.	(f)	4.	(g)
2.	(d)	5.	(b)
3.	(a)	6.	(e)

Items 7 Through 12

(Refer to Table 7-2, page 85)

7.	(f)	10.	(b)
8.	(d)	11.	(c)
9.	(e)	12.	(a)

ANSWERS TO MULTIPLE CHOICE QUESTIONS

Items 1 Through 10

1. (d)   The nurse if promoting independence in Miss H. by explaining how to prepare her insulin injection. Just to give the patient a syringe, needle, and an orange is not helpful; the patient needs to know how to use them correctly. Nurses provide skills, or services, that assist clients to cope with health problems that will not improve. Clients are expected to become actively involved and to retain as much independence as possible.   (81)

2. (c)   The desired outcome of a therapeutic nurse-patient relationship is one of moving toward restoring health.   (81)

3. (a)   The relationship between a patient and a nurse usually begins with a period of getting acquainted. The patient explains health problems that are interfering with the quality of his life. The nurse uses this information to formulate an understanding of the services being sought to help with the problems.   (82)

4. (c)   Verbal communication is communication that uses words. It includes speaking, reading, and writing.   (83)

5. (b)   Nonverbal communication is the exchange of information without using words. It is what is *not* said. People communicate nonverbally through facial expressions, posture, mode of dress, grooming, and movements. Crying, laughing, and moaning are also considered nonverbal communication because they do not use words.   (86)

6. (d)   A common obstacle to effective communication is to ignore the importance of silence.   (85–86)

7. (a)   To promote effective communication, the nurse should avoid "pat" answers that offer false reassurance. These are often misinterpreted by patients as a lack of interest.   (85)

8. (c)   Kinesics refers to body language, or those collective nonverbal techniques like facial expressions, posture, gestures, and body movements.   (86)

9. (a)   Touch is a tactile stimulus produced by making personal contact with another individual. Task-oriented touch involves the personal contact that is required when performing nursing procedures.   (87)

10. (a)   Giving attention to what patients say provides a stimulus for meaningful interaction. It is best to position oneself at the person's level and make frequent eye contact. It is important that the nurse avoid giving signals that indicate impatience, boredom, or the pretense of listening.   (84)

ANSWERS TO TRUE OR FALSE QUESTIONS

Items 1 Through 10

1. *False*. Intimate space is reserved for lovemaking, confiding secrets, sharing confidential information. (See Table 7-3)   (86)
2. *True*.
3. *True*.
4. *False*. Nursing acts are prompted by a concern for the well-being of everyone. (See Display 7-1)   (82)
5. *False*. Identifying the problem, describing desired outcomes, and answering questions honestly are *patient* responsibilities within the nurse-patient relationship. (See Display 7-2)   (82)
6. *True*.
7. *True*.
8. *False*. The introductory phase of the nurse-patient relationship is the period of getting acquainted. The working phase involves mutually planning the patient's care.   (82)
9. *True*.
10. *True*.

ANSWERS TO SHORT ANSWER QUESTIONS

Items 1 Through 3

1. Silence may be used (refer to page 85):
   a. To encourage participation in verbal discussions
   b. To relieve a patient's anxiety by providing a personal presence
   c. to provide a brief period of time to process information
   d. For introspection when needing to explore feelings
   e. To provide an opportunity for prayer
2. Principles providing a basis for a therapeutic relationship include (refer to page 82):
   a. Treating each patient as a unique person
   b. Respecting the patient's feelings
   c. Promoting the patient's physical, emotional, social, and spiritual well-being
   d. Encouraging the patient to participate in problem solving and decision making
   e. Accepting that the patient has the potential for growth and change
3. Touch is a tactile stimulus produced by making personal contact with another individual. Task-oriented touch is the personal contact required to do nursing procedures or provide nursing care. Affective touch is used to demonstrate concern or affection. Affective touch is generally used when the patient is lonesome, uncomfortable, anxious, frightened, or near death. In these situations a hug, a pat on the shoulder, or taking hold of the patient's hand may be examples of affective touch.   (87)

Patient Teaching

The number in parentheses following each rationale indicates on which page in *Fundamental Skills and Concepts in Patient Care,* Seventh Edition, you can find the correct answer.

ANSWERS TO MATCHING QUESTIONS

Items 1 Through 17

(Refer to Table 8-1, page 91)

1. (a)	7. (c)	13. (c)
2. (b)	8. (c)	14. (a)
3. (c)	9. (a)	15. (a)
4. (b)	10. (b)	16. (a)
5. (b)	11. (a)	17. (c)
6. (a)	12. (c)	

Items 18 Through 27

(Refer to Display 8-2, page 90)

18. (b)	23. (a)
19. (c)	24. (b)
20. (a)	25. (c)
21. (b)	26. (b)
22. (a)	27. (a)

ANSWERS TO MULTIPLE CHOICE QUESTIONS

Items 1 Through 15

1. (b) The cognitive domain involves processing information by listening or reading facts and descriptions. (90)
2. (d) The psychomotor domain involves learning by doing. (90)

3. (a) When preparing reading materials for the visually impaired, choose large-size print in black ink on white paper. Letters and words are more distinct when they are set in large print with a typestyle that promotes visual discrimination. Black print on white paper provides maximum contrast and makes the letters more legible. Glossy paper reflects light, causing glare that makes reading more difficult. (92)
4. (c) Hearing loss is generally in the higher-pitch ranges. Select words that do not begin with F, S, or K. These letters are formed with high-pitched sounds and are, therefore, difficult for the hearing impaired person to discriminate. (92)
5. (a) When caring for older adults, it is important to reduce noise and distractions in the environment. (94)
6. (d) Learning is motivated by potential rewards or punishment. (Refer to Table 8-1) (91)
7. (c) The term *literacy* refers to the ability to read and write. (91)
8. (d) Evaluation, the last step in the nursing process, enables nurses to determine whether or not goals have been met. When teaching a skill to a client, the best means of evaluating whether or not the skill has been learned is to observe the client doing the skill. In addition, talking about and doing the injection will assist the client to retain approximately 90% of what was learned. (94)
9. (c) Demonstrating how to do a task involves talking about it and doing it. Learners retain 90% of what they talk about as well as do. (90)
10. (a) Informal teaching is unplanned and occurs spontaneously at the patient's bedside. Formal teaching requires a plan. (93)
11. (d) When the capacity and motivation for learning exist, the final component of learning readiness must be determined. Readiness refers to the pa-

tient's physical and psychological well-being. For example, a person in pain, depressed, or having difficulty breathing is not in the best condition for learning to take place.   (93–94)

12. (b)   Learning a neuromuscular skill is in the psychomotor domain. (See Display 8-2)   (90)

13. (b)   The behaviors associated with the cognitive domain are: list, label, identify, summarize, locate, and select. (See Display 8-2)   (90)

14. (a)   Teaching may be formal if the preplanned information is presented at a scheduled time. Informal teaching occurs spontaneously at the patient's bedside.   (93)

15. (b)   Optimum learning takes place when an individual has a purpose for acquiring new information. The desire for new learning may be to satisfy intellectual curiosity, to restore independence, to prevent complications, or as a means to facilitate discharge and return to the comfort of home. Other, less desirable reasons for learning are to please others and to avoid criticism.   (93)

ANSWERS TO TRUE OR FALSE QUESTIONS

Items 1 Through 10

1. *True.*
2. *False.* Literacy refers to the ability to read and write. Approximately 21% of American adults are illiterate (unable to read or write). Another 27% possess minimal literacy skills (functionally illiterate). Because many of these people are not apt to volunteer this information or they have developed elaborate mechanisms to compensate for their learning deficits, literacy may be difficult to assess.   (91)
3. *True.*
4. *False.* Health teaching is no longer an optional nursing activity. Many nurse practice acts require it, it is required as part of ANA standards, and legal documentation is required in the patient's record.   (89)

5. *True.*
6. *False.* Ceiling lights tend to diffuse light rather than concentrate it on a small area where the patient needs to focus.   (92)
7. *True.*
8. *False.* The desire for new learning may be to satisfy intellectual curiosity, restore independence, prevent complications, or facilitate discharge and return to the comfort of home. Other, less desirable reasons for learning are to please others and to avoid criticism.   (93)
9. *True.*
10. *False.* Because teaching and learning involve language, the nurse must modify teaching approaches if the patient cannot speak English. Language barriers do not justify omitting health teaching.   (92)

ANSWERS TO SHORT ANSWER QUESTIONS

Items 1 and 2

1. Refer to Table 8-1. You may choose any three of those listed for Gerogogic Learners.   (91)
2. Some of the *most* important factors are (refer to pages 89–90):
   a. Style of learning
   b. Developmental stage
   c. Capacity to learn
   d. Motivation for learning
   e. Readiness to learn
   f. What the patient wants to know
   g. What the patient needs to know

CHAPTER 9

Recording and Reporting

The number in parentheses following each rationale indicates on which page in *Fundamental Skills and Concepts in Patient Care*, Seventh Edition, you can find the correct answer.

ANSWERS TO MATCHING QUESTIONS

Items 1 Through 10

(Refer to Table 9-4, page 106)

1. (i)
2. (e)
3. (h)
4. (k)
5. (c)
6. (j)
7. (l)
8. (b)
9. (m)
10. (d)

ANSWERS TO MULTIPLE CHOICE QUESTIONS

Items 1 Through 11

1. (a)   The medical record is a written, chronological account of a person's illness or injury and the health care provided, from the onset of the problem through discharge or death.   (98)
2. (c)   Another purpose of the patient's health record is to ensure safety and continuity in the patient's care. Sharing of information prevents duplication and helps to reduce the chance of error or omission.   (97–98)
3. (d)   Patients' records are admissible as evidence in courts of law in this country. They are the bases for proving or disproving allegations concerning a patient's care. Therefore, it is essential that entries on the records be objectively written, accurate, complete, and legible. (See Display 9-1)   (99)
4. (b)   A traditional record is organized according to the source of information.   (100)
5. (c)   The problem-oriented record is organized according to a patient's specific health problem.   (100)
6. (d)   There are four major parts to a POR. These are the database, the problem list, the initial plan, and the progress notes and follow-up.   (100)
7. (d)   Narrative charting involves writing information about the patient and his care in a chronological order. It is used primarily in traditional records. Each person involved in a patient's care, such as the doctor, nurse, physical therapist, and so on, writes information on separate forms in the patient's chart. This adds bulk to the medical record and tends to fragment the information.   (100)
8. (b)   PIE charting is very similar to a SOAPIER format of charting. "PIE" stands for "problem, intervention, and evaluation." However, when using the PIE method for charting, assessments are documented on a separate form.   (101)
9. (b)   Historically, patients were not allowed to see their health care record. Certain federal laws have now changed that practice. Health agencies have developed guidelines by which patients may read their records.   (100)
10. (a)   3:30 PM is equal to 1530 in military time. To convert to military time, add twelve to every hour after noon. Therefore, by adding 12:00 to 3:30, you get 1530 hours. (See Figure 9-6) (See Table 9-5)   (107)
11. (a)   It is important to write or print clearly when recording a patient's care. Illegible entries on the patient record become questionable information in a court of law. The entry loses its value for exchanging information if it is unreadable.   (99)

ANSWERS TO TRUE OR FALSE QUESTIONS

Items 1 Through 12

1. *True.*
2. *False.* Entries on the patient's health record are made by all health practitioners according to their area of expertise.   (97)
3. *False.* The traditional record is organized according to the source of information. The problem-oriented record is organized according to a patient's specific health problem.   (100)
4. *True.*
5. *False.* Planning, regardless of the way it is recorded, *should always be* done with the patient.   (93)
6. *False.* PIE charting is very similar to a SOAPIER format of charting. However, when using the PIE method for charting, assessments are documented on a separate form.   (101)
7. *False.* Charting by exception is a method of documenting care, but limits the amount of writing to information that is abnormal or deviates from written standards. A checklist is a form that can be used to document routine types of care, such as bathing and mouth care.   (101–102)
8. *True.*
9. *True.*
10. *True.*
11. *True.*
12. *False.* The information on the Kardex should be written in pencil because it is constantly being updated or changed.   (107)

ANSWERS TO SHORT ANSWER QUESTIONS

Items 1 Through 5

(Refer to Table 9-3, page 102)

1. Analysis
2. Evaluation
3. Subjective information
4. Revision
5. Objective information

CHAPTER 10

Admission, Discharge, Transfer, and Referral

The number in parentheses following each rationale indicates on which page in *Fundamental Skills and Concepts in Patient Care,* Seventh Edition, you can find the correct answer.

ANSWERS TO MATCHING QUESTIONS

Items 1 Through 7

(Refer to Table 10-4, page 134)

1. (b)
2. (f)
3. (h)
4. (g)
5. (a)
6. (e)
7. (c)

ANSWERS TO MULTIPLE CHOICE QUESTIONS

Items 1 Through 10

1. (b)   Skilled nursing care involves 24-hour nursing service. A person needing skilled care requires the continuous skills, judgment, and knowledge of a licensed nurse. Exampled of skilled care include caring for wounds, suctioning, tube feeding, and intravenous fluids.   (132)
2. (c)   When the nurse is responsible for handling the patient's valuables and clothing, *the agency's policies must be carefully observed.* It is best to have a second nurse or a representative from the hospital's administrative staff present when a nurse receives valuables for safekeeping. An inventory is sometimes made. The nurse and the patient may cosign the inventory. One copy is given to the patient and the other copy is attached to the chart.   (121)
3. (d)   Referral is often a part of good discharge planning. The nurse should begin to anticipate what kind of care the patient will require before it is time for her to leave. Planning, coordination, and communication take time in order to ensure that patients receive continuity of care.   (134)
4. (b)   Preparing a patient for discharge actually should begin when he is admitted. The purpose of his stay is to help him reach an improved state of wellness, and this begins at the time of admission.   (127)
5. (c)   The patient cannot be forcefully detained when he is a rational adult.   (127)
6. (b)   The nurse responsible for the patient's care should be sure the physician is notified and aware of the patient's wishes to leave. Unsuccessful attempts to locate the doctor should be noted on the patient's record. The hospital's nursing supervisor may also be notified.   (127)
7. (b)   Cleaning a patient's room and equipment after discharge is ordinarily a housekeeping responsibility.   (128)
8. (b)   Early planning helps ensure that continuity of care is maintained. The term means that the patient's care remains uninterrupted despite changes in caregivers, thus avoiding any loss in the progress that has already been made.   (134)
9. (a)   Discharge is a process that occurs when a patient leaves a health agency. It consists of obtaining a written medical order for discharge, completing discharge instructions, notifying the business office, helping the patient leave the health agency, writing a summary of the patient's condition at the time of discharge, and requesting that the room be cleaned.   (126)
10. (b)   Intermediate care facilities provide health-related care and services to individuals who, because of their mental or physical condition, require institutional care but not 24-hour nursing care.   (133)

ANSWERS TO TRUE OR FALSE QUESTIONS

Items 1 Through 10

1. *True.*
2. *True.*
3. *False.* Preparing an identification bracelet for the patient is one of the first components of the admission routine.   (120)
4. *False.* When the nurse learns that a patient will be arriving, the room should be prepared. The patient should feel that everyone on the nursing unit is prepared and ready for his admission.   (120)
5. *True.*
6. *False.* Some hospitals provide booklets with general information for newly admitted patients. Many patients are anxious when they are admitted. Anxiety interferes with the ability to remember. A booklet acts as a reminder for what was explained. Booklets should never take the place of a nurse's explanations.   (121)
7. *False.* Losing personal items belonging to a patient can have serious legal implications for the nurse and the health agency. It is best to have a second nurse or a representative from the hospital's administrative staff present when a nurse receives valuables for safekeeping. An inventory is sometimes made. Problems occur when, in the course of hospitalization, other valuable items are brought in without subsequent documentation.   (121)
8. *True.*
9. *False.* A step-down unit is a special area in the hospital for patients who are recovering from serious conditions, and require less intensive nursing care.   (130)
10. *True.*

ANSWER TO SHORT ANSWER QUESTION

Refer to "Nursing Guidelines For Transferring a Patient" on page 131. You may choose any six actions listed.

CHAPTER 11

Vital Signs

The number in parentheses following each rationale indicates on which page in *Fundamental Skills and Concepts in Patient Care,* Seventh Edition, you can find the correct answer.

ANSWERS TO MATCHING QUESTIONS

Items 1 Through 5

(Refer to Table 11-4, pages 153–154)

1. (b)
2. (f)
3. (d)
4. (e)
5. (a)

Items 6 Through 10

(Refer to Table 11-5, page 156)

6. (c)
7. (f)
8. (b)
9. (a)
10. (d)

Items 11 through 14

(Refer to Table 11-6, page 157)

11. (e)
12. (d)
13. (a)
14. (b)

Items 15 Through 24

(Refer to pages 161 and 163)

15. (d)
16. (f)
17. (h)
18. (c)
19. (o)
20. (j)
21. (a)
22. (g)
23. (n)
24. (b)

ANSWERS TO MULTIPLE CHOICE QUESTIONS

Items 1 Through 24

1. (c)   Body temperature normally remains within a fairly constant range as a result of a balance between heat production and heat loss. This process is regulated by a thermostat-like arrangement in the brain's hypothalamus.   (139)
2. (b)   When the Fahrenheit scale is used, water freezes at 32° F and boils at 212° F.   (138)
3. (a)   The vital signs normally fluctuate in circadian rhythm. The body temperature is ordinarily lowest from midnight to dawn.   (139)
4. (c)   The patient's temperature is 101.8° F. To convert centigrade to Fahrenheit, multiply by 9/5 and add 32. To change Fahrenheit to centigrade, subtract 32 and multiply by 5/9. (Display 11-2, page 139)
5. (c)   Persons having strong emotional experiences, such as fear and anxiety, are likely to have a higher than average temperature. Conversely, persons experiencing apathy and depression are likely to have a lower than average body temperature.   (139)
6. (c)   A patient is considered to be in danger when the temperature reaches beyond 41° C (105.8° F).   (152)
7. (b)   A body temperature below the average normal is called hypothermia.   (155)

8. (c)   Death usually occurs when the temperature falls below approximately 86° F (30° C).   (155)

9. (a)   Cold body temperatures are best measured with a tympanic thermometer.   (155)

10. (a)   Tall, slender persons usually have a slower pulse rate than short, stout persons. The rate for women is slightly faster, by about 7 to 8 beats per minute than it is for men.   (156)

11. (d)   A rapid pulse rate is called tachycardia.   (156)

12. (c)   An irregular pattern of heart beats and consequently an irregular pulse rhythm is called an *arrhythmia*. It may also be called *dysrhythmia*.   (156)

13. (d)   The term *palpitation* means that a person is aware of his or her own heart contraction without having to feel the pulse. The pulse rate is usually rapid when palpitations are noted.   (156)

14. (d)   A rapid and weak pulse is called a thready pulse. This type of pulse is noted when the blood volume is small, making the pulse difficult to feel and, once felt, very easily stopped with pressure.   (156)

15. (d)   The best area to obtain an apical pulse on an adult is at site D. The heart beats are best heard at the apex, or lower tip of the heart. This area is located slightly below the left nipple in line with the middle of the clavicle.   (157)

16. (a)   The difference between the apical and radial pulse rates is called the *pulse deficit*.   (157)

17. (c)   The process of exchanging oxygen and carbon dioxide between the blood and the body is called *internal respiration*. *External respiration* is the process of exchanging oxygen and carbon dioxide between the lungs and the blood.   (161)

18. (b)   The respiratory center in the medulla and specialized sensing tissue in the carotid arteries are very sensitive to the amount of carbon dioxide in the blood.   (161)

19. (c)   The relationship between the pulse and respiratory rates is fairly consistent in normal persons. The ratio is one respiration to approximately 4 or 5 heart beats.   (161)

20. (b)   *Hypoventilation* is a term that describes a less than normal amount of air entering the lungs.   (161)

21. (d)   Blood is pushed forward into the arteries during systole. Systole is the phase during which the heart works. The pressure increases during this time. This is called the *systolic pressure*.   (164)

22. (a)   Blood pressure falls in relation to position changes from lying to sitting or standing. The normal difference in systolic pressure tends to be no greater than 10 mmHg lower than it was in a reclining position.   (174)

23. (a)   The difference between the systolic and diastolic blood pressure measurements is called the pulse pressure. It is computed by subtracting the smaller figure from the larger.   (164)

24. (b)   If the blood pressure cuff is too small, the blood pressure reading will be falsely high.   (165)

ANSWERS TO TRUE OR FALSE QUESTIONS

Items 1 Through 12

1. *False*. Obtaining the apical-radial pulse rate requires two persons. One listens at the apex of the heart while the other feels the pulse at the patient's wrist. They use one watch placed conveniently between them, decide on a specific time to start counting, and count for a full minute.   (157)

2. *True*.

3. *True*.

4. *True*.

5. *True*.

6. *False*. When the nurse assesses a patient for blood pressure changes from lying to upright positions, the patient should be lying for at least 3 minutes.   (173)

7. *False*. The mercury type of sphygmomanometer uses a mercury gauge. The aneroid type does not use mercury but contains a needle that moves about a dial.   (165)

8. *False*. The diastolic pressure cannot be measured using the palpation technique.   (172)

9. *True*.

10. *True*.

11. *True*.

12. *True*.

ANSWERS TO SHORT ANSWER QUESTIONS

Items 1 Through 3

1. Circumstances in which nursing judgment should be used are (refer to pages 165–166):
    a. A change in vital signs is noted and a trend is developing.
    b. Findings are very different from previous recordings.
    c. The vital signs are not in keeping with the patient's condition.
    d. The vital signs could possibly be fraudulent.

2. Refer to Figure 11-14, page 165.

3. Refer to Figure 11-9, page 157.

CHAPTER 12

Physical Assessment

The number in parentheses following each rationale indicates on which page in *Fundamental Skills and Concepts in Patient Care,* Seventh Edition, you can find the correct answer.

ANSWERS TO MATCHING QUESTIONS

Items 1 Through 7

(Refer to chapter 12 text)

1. (d)
2. (f)
3. (h)
4. (a)
5. (g)
6. (e)
7. (c)

Items 8 Through 13

(Refer to Table 12-3, page 193)

8. (d)
9. (f)
10. (a)
11. (e)
12. (g)
13. (b)

ANSWERS TO MULTIPLE CHOICE QUESTIONS

Items 1 Through 10

1. (d) The synonym for rales is crackles. (198)
2. (c) *Inspection* is purposeful observation. Using the term broadly, inspection refers to a technique in which the nurse uses many senses collectively to scan the patient. Using the term more strictly, inspection refers to a technique in which the nurse simultaneously focuses vision and attention looking for minute details. (180)
3. (b) *Palpation* uses the sense of touch to gather information. The examiner feels or presses on the body. (180)
4. (d) *Percussion* is most often used to examine the lungs and abdomen. (180)
5. (c) Patients can be taught to use some assessment methods for detecting certain early signs of disease. Nurses should instruct female patients in the use of inspection and palpation for performing self-breast examinations. (195)
6. (c) Because the trachea is large and close to the mouth, the sound is loud and coarse. (197)
7. (c) Bronchovesicular sounds are heard on either side of the center of the chest and back. They are equal in length during inspiration and expiration with no noticeable pause. (197)
8. (c) A wheal is the skin lesion that is elevated, irregular in shape, and has no free fluid. (See Table 12-4, page 194)
9. (b) A wart is an example of a skin lesion called a papule. (See Table 12-4, page 194)
10. (a) When using percussion to examine a patient, an empty, moderately loud, resonant sound is a normal finding for the lung. (See Table 12-1, page 180)

ANSWERS TO TRUE OR FALSE QUESTIONS

Items 1 Through 10

1. *True.*
2. *False.* The physician also obtains a medical history. Although the data gathered by the physician and the nurse are similar in content, the nurse uses the information differently. Duplication in many areas can be avoided if the nurse is present when the physician obtains the medical history.
3. *False.* Although the patient may have weighed himself recently at home, it is best to weigh him again. The recorded measurements are extremely important in assessing trends in future weight loss or gain and are used to calculate dosages of some drugs.   (182)
4. *True.*
5. *False.* A diseased area of the skin is generally referred to as a lesion. A fissure is a groove or crack in the skin or mucus membrane.   (193)
6. *True.*
7. *True.*
8. *False.* When doing a visual assessment, the nurse should check the six cardinal positions. (188) & Figure 12-14.
9. *False.* Bronchial sounds are heard over the upper portion of the sternum and are harsh and loud.   (197)
10. *True.*

ANSWERS TO SHORT ANSWER QUESTIONS

Items 1 Through 3

1. The recommended techniques for obtaining the patient's height and weight are (refer to pages 182–183):
   a. Check to see that the scale is calibrated to "0."
   b. Ask or assist the patient to remove his robe and shoes if he is wearing them.
   c. Place a paper towel on the scale.
   d. Assist the patient onto the scale.
   e. Slide the weight until the scale balances; read and record the weight.
   f. Ask the patient to stand straight in order to measure the height.
   g. Move the measuring bar down until it lightly touches the top of the patient's head.
   h. Read and record the height.
   i. Record the height and weight on the patient's record.
2. The purposes of a physical assessment are (refer to page 180):
   a. It is an excellent way to evaluate an individual's current health status. It is also a time when health practitioners can teach patients.
   b. It helps detect signs and symptoms of early illness.
   c. Findings contribute to the informational data-based guiding the nursing care that the patient may need.
   d. To evaluate responses to medical and nursing interventions.
3. Techniques to use when assessing the respiratory system are (refer to pages 184, 187–189):
   a. Observe the size and shape of the chest.
   b. Observe the movement of the chest.
   c. Note the type and characteristics of any cough.

CHAPTER 13

Special Examinations and Tests

The number in parentheses following each rationale indicates on which page in *Fundamental Skills and Concepts in Patient Care,* Seventh Edition, you can find the correct answer.

ANSWERS TO MATCHING QUESTIONS

Items 1 Through 5

(Refer to pages 211–212)

1. (g)
2. (d)
3. (a)
4. (e)
5. (c)

Items 6 Through 13

(Refer to chapter 13 text)

6. (b)
7. (f)
8. (c)
9. (e)
10. (a)
11. (g)
12. (h)
13. (d)

ANSWERS TO MULTIPLE CHOICE QUESTIONS

Items 1 Through 12

1. (d)   The suffix *-gram* describes the actual image or results of the test. By combining a root word that refers to a part of the body with a word ending that has a common meaning, the nurse can interpret the definition of medical terms.   (Table 13-1, page 208)

2. (a)   The suffix *-centesis* describes a procedure involving the puncture of a body cavity. A thoracentesis is a puncture of the pleural cavity, which lies in the thorax.   (Table 13-1, page 208)

3. (d)   A *paracentesis* is a procedure that involves puncturing the skin and subsequently the abdominal cavity so that body fluid may be withdrawn.   (225)

4. (a)   Queckenstedt's test is done during a lumbar puncture. This is used to determine the presence or absence of an obstruction to the flow of cerebrospinal fluid.   (226)

5. (c)   Electroencephalography is an examination that records an image of the electrical activity in the brain. It is abbreviated EEG.   (224)

6. (b)   The dorsal recumbent position is used most often to examine the rectum and vagina.   (Table 13-2, page 211)

7. (d)   The lithotomy position is used to examine the vagina with a speculum. It is also used when the internal female reproductive organs are palpated, and when male or female bladder inspections are done with a cystoscope.   (See Table 13-2, page 211)

8. (d)   In some cases, a signed consent form may be required before certain tests or examinations may be performed. In order to be legally sound, consent must contain three elements: capacity, comprehension, and voluntariness.   (See Display 13-2, page 209)

9. (d)   A cystoscopy refers to an examination that involves inspection of the urinary bladder.   (See Display 13-4, page 220)

10. (c)   The modified standing position is most commonly used to examine the prostate gland.   (See Table 13-2, page 212)

11. (b)   A Class III result on the cellular portion of the Pap smear indicates that the sample on the smear is suggestive of cancer cells, but is not definite.   (See Table 13-3, page 213)

12. (a) A #1 result on the identifiable microorganisms portion of the Pap smear indicates that the sample contained normal microorganisms. (See Table 13-3, page 213)

ANSWERS TO TRUE OR FALSE QUESTIONS

Items 1 Through 15

1. *True.*
2. *False.* Many examinations and tests require special preparation of the patient in order to obtain accurate results. The requirements for certain tests are usually located in a reference manual at each nursing unit. The nurse should refer to these written instructions each time a patient is undergoing a test *rather than rely on memory.* (209)
3. *True.*
4. *False. Draping* is a term that refers to covering a body part in such a manner that it does not interfere with access to the area being examined. Draping avoids exposing the patient unnecessarily. If the patient feels chilled, a sheet or blanket may be used to cover him. (210)
5. *True.*
6. *False.* The atomic structure of some chemical elements, such as iodine, can be altered in such a way that it gives off radiation. It is then referred to as a *radionuclide.* (220)
7. *True.*
8. *True.*
9. *True.*
10. *False.* Unless alcohol evaporates before the finger stick, it can alter the results. (231)
11. *True.*
12. *True.*
13. *False.* Glucose is the type of sugar present in the blood as a result of eating carbohydrates. Normal blood levels are maintained by the body's production of glucagons and insulin, hormones that regulate glucose metabolism. (228)
14. *True.*
15. *True.*

ANSWERS TO SHORT ANSWER QUESTIONS

Items 1 Through 3

1. Items to record on the patient's record include (refer to page 213):
   a. The date and time
   b. Pertinent pre-examination assessments and preparation
   c. The type of examination or test
   d. Who performed the test and where it was done
   e. The patient's responses during and after the procedure
   f. The type of specimen that was collected (i.e., tissue, fluid, blood)
   g. A description of the specimen (i.e., size, appearance, volume, color) and from where it was taken
   h. The disposition of the specimen
2. Factors to be considered when procedures are done on older adults are: (229)
   a. Unless separate age-specific norms are available, test findings from older adults may be misinterpreted.
   b. Prescription drugs may affect test results.
   c. Check with the physician before giving multiple daily medications (with a small amount of water) to older adults who are fasting for a procedure.
   d. Older adults may not be able to tolerate having food and fluids withheld for long periods of time.
   e. Dehydration may cause blood values to seem elevated.
   f. Intensive and repeated bowel preparation for some tests may cause exhaustion.
   g. A bedside commode and assistance to use it is a frequent need for older adults.
   h. A bed alarm that sounds when the patient gets out of bed may be a necessary safety precaution for older adults who need assistance to the bathroom or bedside commode.
   i. Coordinate tests and examinations to diminish waiting time and extensive preparation and provide increased periods of rest.
   j. It may be appropriate to warm blankets, slippers, and robes if the older adult has to wait in drafty or air-conditioned hallways.
   k. After the procedure, offer food, fluid, and an opportunity to use the toilet, and then allow for rest before beginning other nursing activities.

3. Patient responsibilities prior to out-patient procedures include (refer to page 209):
   a. If questions, call (provide a number for the patient to call).
   b. Do *not* eat or drink anything for at least 8 to 12 hours prior to the test.
   c. Follow all dietary restrictions or recommendations for the procedure.
   d. Check with your physician about taking regular medications on the day of the procedure.
   e. Bathe or shower as usual.
   f. Dress casually and comfortably in layers.
   g. Ask a friend or family member to bring you to the examination and take your home after.
   h. Come to the test or examination location at least one-half hour before the scheduled time.
   i. Check in at the _____ desk when you arrive.
   j. Bring insurance information and/or forms with you.
   k. Bring a list of medications you take and a list of your allergies with you.

CHAPTER 14

Nutrition

The number in parentheses following each rationale indicates on which page in *Fundamental Skills and Concepts in Patient Care,* Seventh Edition, you can find the correct answer.

ANSWERS TO MATCHING QUESTIONS

Items 1 Through 5

(Refer to Table 14-2, page 242)

1. (d)
2. (f)
3. (b)
4. (g)
5. (e)

Items 6 Through 8

(Refer to Table 14-3, page 243)

6. (c)
7. (d)
8. (b)

Items 9 Through 13

(Refer to page 254)

9. (c)
10. (g)
11. (a)
12. (d)
13. (f)

ANSWERS TO MULTIPLE CHOICE QUESTIONS

Items 1 Through 16

1. (b) Nutrition is defined as the process whereby the body uses food. (239)
2. (d) A calorie is the amount of heat necessary to raise the temperature of 1 gram of water 1° C. (240)
3. (c) Most average adults need between 2000 and 3000 calories per day according to the National Research Council of the National Academy of Science. (240)
4. (a) Proteins are the source of amino acids. (240)
5. (d) Fats have a higher energy value than other nutrients; they yield 9 calories per gram. (240)
6. (c) The Department of Health and Human Resources in its publication, *Healthy People 2000: National Health Promotion and Disease Prevention Objectives* (1992), has recommended that Americans reduce their present fat intake to no more than 30% of their daily calories. (241)
7. (c) Minerals, such as calcium, sodium, potassium, and chloride, are chemical substances. When these substances are dissolved in the body, they are called electrolytes. (242)
8. (a) Those who arbitrarily select to become vegetarians may need to learn how to combine plant sources to ensure that they are consuming adequate amounts of all the essential amino acids. (245)
9. (c) Regurgitation occurs quite commonly among infants after eating. (252)
10. (a) Offer a light but nutritious breakfast. Often, the condition worsens during the day, but the appetite may be good for the first meal of the day. (252)

11. (b)   Low-density lipoproteins transport cholesterol to cells and tissue.   (See Table 14-1, page 241)

12. (c)   Very low-density lipoproteins become a major source of low-density lipoproteins. (See Table 14-1, page 241)

13. (d)   The normal range of measurement for the triceps skin fold in adult males is 12.5–7.3 mm.   (See Table 14-4, page 249)

14. (a)   Minerals are noncaloric substances in food that are essential to all cells.   (229)

15. (a)   The term *dysphagia* means difficulty swallowing.   (254)

16. (c)   Good sources of carbohydrates include cereals and grains, such as rice, wheat and wheat germ, oats, barley, corn and corn meal, fruits and vegetables, molasses, maple and corn syrups, honey, and common table sugar.   (241)

ANSWERS TO TRUE OR FALSE QUESTIONS

Items 1 Through 10

1. *False.* Most eating habits are learned in early life and vary from culture to culture.   (244)

2. *False. Anorexia* is the loss of appetite or lack of desire for food. *Cachexia* is a condition in which there is a general wasting away of body tissue.   (251)

3. *True.*

4. *True.*

5. *False.* Protein complementation is the act of combining two or more plant sources in the same meal.   (240)

6. *True.*

7. *False.* Many deficiency diseases have been associated with diets in which specific foods, rich in a source of *a vitamin,* have been lacking.   (241)

8. *False. Fat-soluble* vitamins are stored in reserve in the body for future needs.   (242)

9. *True.*

10. *True*

ANSWERS TO SHORT ANSWER QUESTIONS

Items 1 Through 2

1. According to the food pyramid, the food groups and their daily servings are (refer to Figure 14-2, page 232):
   a. Bread, cereal, rice, pasta   6–11 servings
   b. Vegetables   3–5 servings
   c. Fruits   2–4 servings
   d. Milk, yogurt, cheese   2–3 servings
   e. Meat, poultry, fish, eggs, beans, nuts   2–3 servings
   f. Fats, oils, sweets   Use sparingly

2. Facts that appear on a nutritional label are (refer to text and Figure 14-3, page 247):
   a. Serving size
   b. Number of servings in container
   c. Calories per serving
   d. Number of calories from fat
   e. Total fat
   f Amount of saturated fat
   g. Cholesterol
   h. Amount of sodium
   i. Total carbohydrate
      1. Dietary fiber
      2. Sugars
   j. Protein
   k. Vitamins and minerals, if any
   l. Percent of daily value based on 2000- and 2500-calorie diet
   m. Number of calories per gram for fat, carbohydrate, and protein
   n. Percent of daily value supplied by each nutrient present in each serving contained in the container

CHAPTER 15

Fluid and Chemical Balance

The number in parentheses following each rationale indicates on which page in *Fundamental Skills and Concepts in Patient Care*, Seventh Edition, you can find the correct answer.

ANSWERS TO MATCHING QUESTIONS

Items 1 Through 6

(Refer to Table 15-2, page 265)

1. (c)	4. (a)
2. (d)	5. (e)
3. (f)	6. (b)

Items 7 Through 12

(Refer to Table 15-7, page 292)

7. (c)	10. (f)
8. (e)	11. (d)
9. (b)	12. (a)

Items 13 Through 19

(Refer to Table 15-9, page 305)

13. (f)	17. (e)
14. (c)	18. (d)
15. (g)	19. (b)
16. (a)	

ANSWERS TO MULTIPLE CHOICE QUESTIONS

Items 1 Through 35

1. (c) The human body is composed of approximately 45% to 75% water. The amount varies according to an individual's age, gender, and body fat composition. (264)

2. (d) The infant would have the most body water. (See Table 15-1, page 264)

3. (a) The total amount of water that adults consume each day is about 1200 to 1500 ml. An additional 700 to 100 ml per day is extracted from the foods eaten. As a result of metabolism, about 200 to 400 ml per day is added to the total fluid intake to bring it to about 2100 to 2900 ml per day. (See Table 15-3, page 266)

4. (b) Most of the water is lost through the kidneys. Some moisture is lost in the stool and in obvious perspiration from areas where skin contains abundant sweat glands. A certain amount of water is lost in a form that cannot usually be seen or felt. This is called insensible water loss. It occurs from the lungs during expiration and through the skin. (See Table 15-3, page 266)

5. (b) Body fluid is located in two general compartments: inside and outside cells. The fluid inside the cells is referred to as intracellular fluid. (264)

6. (c) Osmosis is a process that regulates the distribution of water from one compartment to another. Under the influence of osmosis, water moves through a semipermeable membrane from an area where the fluid is more dilute to another area where the fluid is more concentrated. (265)

7. (c) One of the simplest methods for objectively assessing fluid balance is to compare the amount of a patient's fluid intake with fluid output. (267)

8. (a) When an individual is healthy, the amount of fluid that is taken in should approximate the same amount that is lost. (267)

9. (b) In some cases, the ensure accurate assessment of fluid loss, the nurse may be required to measure liquid stool or weigh wet linens, diapers, or dressings saturated with blood or other secretions. The weight of wet items is compared to the weight of a similar dry item. An estimate of output is based on the knowledge that one pint (475 ml) of water weighs about 1 pound (0.47 kg). (269)

10. (c) The skin may appear warm, flushed, and dry when the patient is experiencing fluid deficit. It may appear cool, pale, and moist in fluid excess. (See Table 15-4, page 267)

11. (b) *Fluid imbalance* is a general term describing any of several conditions in which the body water is not in proper volume or location within the body. One of the locations in which fluid levels is likely to become imbalanced is the blood, or the area of intravascular fluid. When fluid is excessive in this location, the term *hypervolemia* is used to describe it. This term means that there is a high volume, or amount, of water present in the blood.   (273)

12. (d) Fluid imbalance can occur when fluid becomes trapped in interstitial areas. This is called *third spacing*. It often occurs when there is a loss of proteins from the plasma of blood.   (274)

13. (c) Intravenous solutions are selected and ordered by the physician. They are considered to be a form of medication. The specific type of solution, volume, and rate of administration is part of the medical order. The nurse must exercise extreme caution that the correct solution is infused. This is a priority concern because any substance that is instilled directly into the circulatory system produces a rapid effect, due to its almost instant distribution throughout the body.   (277)

14. (d) Intravenous fluids fall into two basic categories. They are either a crystalloid or a colloid solution. A crystalloid solution is a mixture of water and uniformly dissolved crystals, such as salt and sugar.   (275)

15. (b) Crystalloid solutions are further subdivided into isotonic, hypotonic, and hypertonic solutions on the basis of the amount of dissolved crystals present in the solution. A hypotonic solution contains fewer crystals than normally found in plasma. When infused intravenously, the water in the solution will enter through the semipermeable membrane of blood cells. The blood cells will become larger as they fill with water.   (276)

16. (c) A hypertonic solution has a higher amount of dissolved crystals than plasma. It will draw water into the intravascular compartment from the more dilute areas of water within the cells and interstitial spaces. This can help relieve edema because cells and tissues shrink and dehydrate from fluid loss.   (276)

17. (c) Normally, the pressure in the patient's vein is higher than atmospheric pressure. The solution is placed on a standard at a level of 45 to 60 cm   (18 to 24 inches) above the level of the vein. At this height,

gravity is sufficient to overcome the pressure within the vein and allow the solution to infuse.   (276)

18. (d) For most intravenous infusions for adults, an 18, 20, or 22 gauge needle is used. A size 18 or 20 gauge needle should be selected when colloid solutions are infused because a smaller needle may become plugged with the suspended proteins.   (289)

19. (c) Superficial veins are more easily located and are more accessible for puncturing. Veins in the arms and hands are used in preference to veins in the foot or leg. Use veins in the arm or hand on the patient's nondominant side. In general, when the arm is used, it is *best* to select a vein as low as possible on the back of the hand or the lower forearm.   (283)

20. (c) A common time frame for changing an intravenous solution is every 24 hours or when it is finished.   (293)

21. (b) A common practice is to change the dressing over the venipuncture site once in every 24 to 72 hours.   (293)

22. (a) Swelling in the area of the venipuncture site and coolness of the skin are two of the signs of infiltration. The other signs of infiltration include slowing or stopping of the flow and discomfort.   (292)

23. (c) The first nursing action when discontinuing an intravenous infusion is to clamp the tubing and remove the tape that held the dressing and venipuncture device in place.   (296)

24. (b) Dextran is a plasma expander.   (277)

25. (d) A scalp vein is often used for an infant.   (283)

26. (c) Nonelectrolytes are chemical compounds that remain bound together when dissolved in a solution and, therefore, cannot conduct electricity. Glucose is an example of a nonelectrolyte.   (265)

27. (a) Electrolytes are chemical compounds that dissolve and separate into individual molecules, each carrying either a positive or negative electrical charge. In general, these separated molecules are called *ions*. More specifically, a *cation* is an ion with a positive electrical charge. An *anion* is an ion with a negative electrical charge.   (264)

28. (c) Electrolytes are distributed in different proportions in extracellular and intracellular tissue. Their proportions remain relatively constant due to the movement and relocation of various ions through the processes of diffusion and active transport. *Diffusion* is the process in which ions move from an area of greater concentration to an area of lesser concentration through a semipermeable membrane.   (266)

29. (b) Active transport is a process requiring energy in order to move molecules through a semipermeable membrane from an area of low concentration to one that is higher. Diffusion acts passively, with no release of energy. (266)

30. (d) Potassium is a cation. It is the most abundant cation in intracellular fluid. (Table 15-2, page 265)

31. (b) A medication lock is a sealed chamber that is inserted into a venipuncture device. (297)

32. (c) The term *parenteral nutrition* refers to a technique for providing nutrients, such as protein, carbohydrate, fat, vitamins, minerals, and trace elements, intravenously rather than orally. (304)

33. (a) Peripheral parenteral nutrition is an isotonic or hypotonic nutrient solution that provides temporary nutritional support when oral intake is expected to resume in 7 to 10 days. (304)

34. (d) Total parenteral nutrition is a hypertonic solution of nutrients that provide a method of introducing nourishment through either the subclavian or jugular vein directly into the heart via the superior vena cava. (305)

35. (c) An emulsion is a mixture of two liquids, one of which is insoluable in the other, but when combined is distributed throughout as small droplets within the other. A lipid emulsion is a mixture of water and fats in the form of soybean or safflower oil, egg yolk, phospholipids, and glycerin. (306)

ANSWERS TO TRUE OR FALSE QUESTIONS

Items 1 Through 20

1. *False.* A *cation* is an electrolyte with a positive charge. An *anion* is an electrolyte with a negative charge. (264)

2. *False. Diffusion* is a process in which dissolved substances move passively through a semipermeable membrane from an area of higher concentration to an area of lower concentration. *Osmosis* is the movement of water through a semipermeable membrane from an area of lower concentration of dissolved substances to one of higher concentration. (266)

3. *True.*

4. *False.* The extracellular fluid is subdivided into intravascular fluid and interstitial fluid. (264)

5. *True.*

6. *False.* Most of the water in the body is lost through the kidneys. Insensible water loss is the water that is lost through the skin and lungs. (266)

7. *True.*

8. *False.* When the amount of a liquid is not known, a calibrated pitcher should be used to measure the volume. The nurse should avoid estimating an amount. Too often the estimate is inaccurate. (269)

9. *False.* Fluid output is the sum of all the liquid eliminated from the body. Fluid output is determined by measuring urine, emesis, drainage from tubes, and fluid drained following irrigation. (269)

10. *True.*

11. *False.* The skin may appear warm, flushed, and dry when the patient is experiencing fluid deficit. It may appear cool, pale, and moist in fluid excess. (267)

12. *False.* The consumption of salty food can affect the intake and retention of fluids.

13. *True.*

14. *False.* Sodium is the most common electrolyte in the extracellular fluid. (265)

15. *True.*

16. *False.* A glass container of solution requires vented tubing. Because a plastic bag collapses upon itself while the solution infuses, unvented tubing can be used. (278)

17. *True.*

18. *False.* An angiocath is a flexible catheter threaded *over* a needle into a vein. An intracath is a flexible catheter threaded *through* a needle into a vein. (283–284)

19. *True.*

20. *False.* Crossmatching is a laboratory test that determines whether blood specimens of the donor and the recipient are compatible. *Typing* is the laboratory test that identifies the proteins on red blood cells. (301)

ANSWERS TO SHORT ANSWER QUESTIONS

Items 1 Through 5

1. Factors to be considered when selecting a vein for intravenous infusion are (refer to page 284–285):
   a. Superficial veins are more easily located and more accessible.
   b. Veins in the arms and hands are preferred to veins in the foot and lower leg. The circulation may be reduced in the lower extremities.
   c. The patient is less likely to be inconvenienced if the veins on the nondominant side are used.
   d. Choices may be limited due to other factors, such as injury to or surgery on the upper extremities.
   e. Avoid compromising joint movement.
   f. Use the veins far down on the arm and hand first so that if problems arise, there are others available farther up the forearm.
   g. Use a vein that is fairly straight.

h. Avoid thin-walled and scarred veins.

i. Avoid inserting the needle into a valve of the vein.

j. Use larger veins for hypertonic solutions, those containing irritating medications, those administered rapidly, and those that are thick and sticky.

k. Consider the future need for veins and use care in the selection.

2. Steps for cleansing the venipuncture site include (refer to Skill 15-3, page 287):

a. Use betadine or alcohol to cleanse the skin.

b. Start at center of site and cleanse in a circular motion outward 2 to 4 inches.

c. Allow antiseptic to dry.

3. The signs of complications that may occur when a patient is receiving intravenous fluids are (refer to Table 15-7, page 292):

a. *Circulatory overload:* Check for signs and symptoms of dyspnea, noisy respirations, and coughing, possibly caused by too rapid administration.

b. *Infiltration:* Check for swelling of the tissues, pallor and coldness of the skin at the site, complaints of burning sensations, and slowing or stopping of the flow.

c. *Phlebitis:* Check for redness, warmth, and swelling. The patient may complain of pain or burning in the area of the venipuncture site.

d. *Infection:* Check for all of the above signs in addition to purulent drainage from the venipuncture site.

e. *Air embolism:* Caused by air entering the circulatory system—the patient will experience a sudden drop in blood pressure, tachycardia, cyanosis, and a diminished level of consciousness.

4. Refer to Table 15-6, page 276.

Blood Product	Purpose for Administration
a. Platelets	Restore or improve ability to control bleeding
b. Granulocytes	Improve ability to overcome infection
c. Plasma	Replace clotting factors; increase intravascular fluid volume
d. Albumin	Pull third-spaced fluid by increasing colloidal osmotic pressure
e. Cryoprecipitate	Treat blood-clotting disorders

5. Techniques for promoting vein distension are (refer to Display 15-4, page 285):

a. Apply a tourniquet or blood pressure cuff tightly about the arm.

b. Have the patient make a fist and pump the fist intermittently.

c. Tap the skin over the vein several times.

d. Lower the patient's arm to promote distal pooling of blood.

e. Stroke the skin in the direction of the fingers.

f. Apply warm compresses for ten minutes; then reapply the tourniquet.

Hygiene

The number in parentheses following each rationale indicates on which page in *Fundamental Skills and Concepts in Patient Care,* Seventh Edition, you can find the correct answer.

ANSWERS TO MATCHING QUESTIONS

Items 1 through 6

(Refer to pages 313, 329, and 332)

1. (d)
2. (e)
3. (b)
4. (c)
5. (g)
6. (a)

Items 7 through 10

(Refer to Table 16-4, page 332)

7. (c)
8. (e)
9. (b)
10. (f)

ANSWERS TO MULTIPLE CHOICE QUESTIONS

Items 1 Through 14

1. (b)   The primary concern for nurses is that hygiene be carried out in a manner that promotes health. The other choices may or may not be of concern for the nurse.   (311)
2. (d)   The main component of the integumentary system is the skin.   (312)
3. (a)   Many bacteria in the mouth become lodged between the teeth. The toothbrush cannot reach these areas well. Therefore, flossing several times a day is recommended. Flossing helps to break up groups of bacteria between the teeth.   (328)
4. (b)   Soak the feet of the patient before trimming brittle, thick toenails.   (333)
5. (d)   If the hair is tangled, use a wide-toothed comb and comb starting at the ends of the hair rather than from the crown downward.   (333)
6. (a)   Sudoriferous glands in the skin regulate body temperature. (See Table 16-1, page 313)
7. (c)   Immersion of the buttocks and perineum in a small basin of continuously circulating water is called a sitz bath. (See Table 16-2, page 314)
8. (b)   Many substances may be used for mouth care. Milk of magnesia reduces oral acidity, dissolves plaque, increases the flow of saliva, and soothes oral lesions. (See Table 16-4, page 332)
9. (d)   The accumulation of cerumen within the ear may cause reduced or absent sound from a hearing aid. (See Table 16-5, page 338)
10. (a)   The temperature of the water for a tub bath should be between 105 and 110° F. (See Skill 16-1)   (315)
11. (c)   The skin consists of the epidermis, dermis, and subcutaneous layers. The epidermis, or outermost layer, contains dead skin cells that form a tough protein called keratin, which serves to protect the underlying layers and structures within the skin.   (312)
12. (a)   The teeth begin to erupt at about 6 months of age and continue to do so for 2 or 2 1/2 more years.   (313)
13. (d)   Gingivitis is an inflammation of the gums.   (313)

14. (c)   A partial bath consists of washing those areas of the body that are subject to the greatest soiling or sources of body odor, such as the face, hands, and axillae. Partial bathing may be done at a sink or with a basin at the bedside.   (317)

ANSWERS TO TRUE OR FALSE QUESTIONS

Items 1 Through 12

1. *False.* Some patients wear eyeglasses in addition to their contact lenses. For this reason the nurse should not assume that a patient who wears eyeglasses does not use at least one contact lens.   (336)
2. *False.* Generally, routine hygiene measures are documented on a checklist. (Skill 16-1, page 317)
3. *True.*
4. *False.* Consult with the patient to determine personal preferences. This promotes cooperation between the patient and nurse and allows patient participation in decision making. (Skill Procedures, 301)
5. *True.*
6. *False.* Plain water is most often used to cover dentures when they are not in the mouth, you may add mouthwash or denture cleanser to the water.   (333)
7. *True.*
8. *False.* Preparations made with oil should be used on dry hair. Alcohol is suggested for loosening some tangles.   (333)
9. *True.*
10. *False.* Sebaceous glands located within the hair follicles release an oily substance called sebum.   (312)
11. *True.*
12. *True.*

ANSWERS TO SHORT ANSWER QUESTIONS

Items 1 Through 4

1. The functions of the skin are   (312)
   a. Protects the body
   b. Helps regulate body temperature
   c. Assists with the body's fluid and chemical balance
   d. Has nerve endings that are sensitive to pain, temperature, touch, and pressure
   e. Produces vitamin D with the help of sunlight, and the vitamin D is then absorbed from the skin into the body
2. The characteristics of healthy nails are (refer to page 313):
   a. Thin
   b. Pink
   c. Smooth
   d. A free white margin should extend from the end of each nail
   e. The skin around the nail should be intact
3. Adults normally have 32 teeth.   (313)
4. The reasons for bathing are (refer to pages 313–314):
   a. It cleans and refreshes.
   b. Warm water and massage associated with washing and drying aid in relaxation.
   c. It stimulates circulation.
   d. It reduces the chance for infection.
   e. It may help self-image and morale.
   f. It eliminates body odor.

CHAPTER 17

Comfort, Rest, and Sleep

The number in parentheses following each rationale indicates on which page in *Fundamental Skills and Concepts in Patient Care,* Seventh Edition, you can find the correct answer.

ANSWERS TO MATCHING QUESTIONS.

Items 1 Through 6

(Refer to Table 17-5, page 367)

1. (f)
2. (d)
3. (a)
4. (c)
5. (b)
6. (e)

Items 7 through 11

(Refer to Table 17-1, page 356)

7. (c)
8. (e)
9. (d)
10. (a)
11. (b)

ANSWERS TO MULTIPLE CHOICE QUESTIONS

Items 1 Through 20

1. (b)   For sleep to occur, the individual must be relaxed.   (Table 17-3, page 357)
2. (d)   Phenomena that cycle on a daily basis are referred to as circadian rhythms.   (356)
3. (c)   Sleep is a basic human need characterized by a state of arousable unconsciousness.   (341)
4. (a)   REM sleep is the phase in which most dreaming occurs.   (Table 17-1, 356)
5. (d)   If the onset of sleep is delayed more than 20 to 30 minutes, get out of bed and do something else, like reading.   (360)
6. (c)   Blue and colors with blue tints, such as mauve and light green, promote relaxation.   (342)
7. (c)   Most patients are comfortable when the room temperature is 68° to 74° F (20° to 23° C).   (342)
8. (b)   The REM phase of sleep is referred to as paradoxical sleep because the EEG waves appear similar to those produced during periods of wakefulness, but it is the *deepest* stage of sleep. REM is active sleep. Darting eye movements occur.   (356)
9. (a)   Refer to table 17-1   (356)
10. (c)   In the absence of bright light, the pineal gland secretes melatonin. Light triggers the suppression of melatonin.   (356)
11. (d)   The photoperiod is the number of daylight hours to which a person is accustomed.   (361)
12. (b)   The symptoms of seasonal affective disorder begin during the darker winter months and disappear in the spring.   (361)
13. (d)   Tryptophan is found in protein foods and dairy products.   (357)
14. (b)   Narcolepsy is a sleep disorder characterized by the sudden onset of daytime sleep.   (360)
15. (a)   Newborns sleep approximately 16–20 hours per day.   (Table 17-2, 356).
16. (d)   Five and six-year-olds spend 20% of their sleep in REM sleep.   (Table 17-2, 356)
17. (d)   In severe cases of sleep apnea, patients wear a special breathing mask that keeps the alveoli inflated at all times.   (360)

18. (d)   Parasomnias are non-life-threatening activities that cause arousal or partial arousal, usually during transitions in NREM periods of sleep. (361)
19. (a)   Restless legs syndrome is also known as nocturnal myoclonus. (361)
20. (a)   Sundown Syndrome in older adults is characterized by disorientation as the sun sets. (Display 17-4, 368)

ANSWERS TO TRUE OR FALSE QUESTIONS

Items 1 Through 10

1. *True.*
2. *True.*
3. *True.*
4. *False.* NREM sleep usually precedes REM sleep, the phase during which most dreaming occurs. (356)
5. *False.* The indoor lighting under which most shift workers are exposed is not bright enough to adequately suppress melatonin. Consequently, many shift workers fight to stay awake. According to recent research, most individuals who work night shifts never completely adapt to the reversal of day and night activities no matter how long the pattern is established. (361)
6. *True.*
7. *True.*
8. *True.*
9. *False.* Tranquilizers are drugs that produce a relaxing and calming effect. *Hypnotics* are drugs that induce sleep. (358)
10. *False.* Sleep apnea is highest among older adults, especially obese men who snore. (360)

ANSWERS TO SHORT ANSWER QUESTIONS

Items 1 Through 3

1. Components of phototherapy used to relieve the symptoms of seasonal affective disorder include (Refer to Display 17-3, page 361):
    a. Initiate a schedule of full-spectrum light exposure in October or November.
    b. Remove eye glasses or contact lenses that have ultraviolet filters.
    c. Sit within three feet of light source for 2 hours.
    d. Glance at light periodically. May do other things like read.
    e. Repeat exposure to light after sundown.
    f. Cumulative exposure is 3 to 6 hours/day.
    g. Continue light exposure until spring.
2. Tips for patient teaching to promote sleep include (refer to Patient Teaching for Promoting Sleep, page 360):
    a. Take diuretics early in the morning.
    b. Exercise regularly during the day but not late in the evening.
    c. Don't nap during the day.
    d. Avoid alcohol, nicotine, and caffeine.
    e. Eat dairy products and other proteins daily.
    f. Modify temperature and ventilation to your preference.
    g. Use the bedroom just for sleeping.
    h. Maintain personal sleep rituals.
    i. Use ear plugs and eye shades.
    j. Maintain consistent sleep routines.
    k. If not asleep in 20 to 30 minutes, get out of bed and do something else.
    l. Avoid sleeping medications unless ordered by a physician.
    m. Follow labeled directions on any medications.
3. Tips for patient teaching related to facilitating the use of progressive relaxation include (refer to Nursing Guidelines for Facilitating Progressive Relaxation, page 362):
    a. Select a quiet, dimly lit, private room.
    b. Assume a comfortable lying or sitting position.
    c. Avoid talking.
    d. Close your eyes and focus on breathing.
    e. Inhale deeply through the nose, exhale slowly out the mouth.
    f. Tighten a group of muscles (i.e., left arm or right foot) and hold for five seconds.
    g. Relax those muscles and focus on the pleasurable feeling.
    h. Continue doing steps f and g above until all muscle groups have been exercised and relaxed.
    i. During the exercises, focus on how relaxed you feel and notice the feeling of weightlessness you experience.
    j. Count from 10 to 1 as you begin to move about ending this period of progressive relaxation.

CHAPTER 18

Safety

The number in parentheses following each rationale indicates on which page in *Fundamental Skills and Concepts in Patient Care,* Seventh Edition, you can find the correct answer.

ANSWERS TO MATCHING QUESTIONS

Items 1 Through 10

(Refer to Chapter 19 text)

1. (j)
2. (e)
3. (h)
4. (i)
5. (b)

ANSWERS TO MULTIPLE CHOICE QUESTIONS

Items 1 Through 12

1. (b)   The content of a Class B fire extinguisher is carbon dioxide.   (Table 18-3, page 376)
2. (d)   When a fire occurs, the first measure the nurse should follow is to evacuate the people in the room with the fire. Remembering the shortened version of the steps as *RACE* will help the nurse *Rescue* the people first before *A,* giving the alarm; *C,* confining the fire; and *E,* extinguishing the fire.   (375)
3. (c)   When an accident does occur, check the patient's condition immediately. Note his condition and be ready to describe it accurately.   (389)
4. (b)   After the patient is properly cared for and the physician notified, prepare an incident or accident report. All information related to the accident is entered on the form. It is signed by the person completing the form.   (399)
5. (c)   A *thermal burn,* which is the most common, is a type of skin injury caused by flames, hot liquids, or steam. Burns may also result from contact with caustic chemicals, electric wires, or lightning.   (374)
6. (a)   Asphyxiation is a term that means the inability to breathe.   (376)
7. (d)   The body is quite susceptible to electrical shock because it is composed of water and electrolytes, both of which are good conductors of electricity. A conductor is a substance that facilitates the flow of electrical current.   (377)
8. (b)   Falls, more than any other injury discussed thus far, are the most prevalent accident experienced by older adults, and they have the most serious consequences for this age group.   (378)
9. (d)   The National Fire Protection Association recommends using the acronym RACE, which stands for: R = Rescue; A = Alarm; C = Confine (the fire); and E = Extinguish to identify the essential steps in fire rescues proceedings.   (375)
10. (a)   Macroshock, if it occurs, is the harmless distribution of low-amperage electricity over a large area of the body. Macroshock is experienced as a slight tingling.   (377)
11. (c)   There are Class A, B, C, and ABC fire extinguishers. Class A extinguishers are used for paper, wood, and cloth fires.   (Table 18-3, page 376)
12. (a)   Although physical restraints prevent falls, they create concomitant risks for constipation, incontinence, more infections like pneumonia, pressure sores, and a progressive decline in the ability to perform activities of daily living.   (380)

ANSWERS TO TRUE OR FALSE QUESTIONS

Items 1 Through 10

1. *True.*
2. *False.* It is best to place *moist* blankets on the threshold to contain smoke.   (375)
3. *True.*
4. *True.*
5. *False.* Victims of cold-water drownings are more apt to be resuscitated because of their lowered metabolism, which conserves oxygen, than those who succumb in warm water.   (377)
6. *False.* Poisonings are more prevalent in homes than in health care institutions. More often than not, accidental poisonings occur among toddlers and usually involve the ingestion of substances that are located in the bathroom or kitchen. This is not to imply that poisonings never occur in health care institutions. One could consider medication errors in which the wrong medication or dose is administered to the wrong patient a form of poisoning.   (377)
7. *False.* Educating children is not the only way to prevent childhood poisoning, although it certainly is one component.   (378)
8. *True.*
9. *True.*
10. *False.* Among older adults, hospitalizations are twice as lengthy for those who fall as compared to those who do not, and about half of those who are hospitalized for falling eventually become transferred to a nursing home.   (389)

ANSWERS TO SHORT ANSWER QUESTIONS

Items 1 Through 5

1. Applying a restraint without just cause or a medical order could result in being sued for false imprisonment. Consulting with a doctor or a nursing supervisor helps collaborate that this is the most reasonable action to protect the patient.   (380–381)
2. Methods for helping to prevent falls are (refer to Chapter 18 text):
   a. Place adjustable beds in low position when patients are getting in and out of bed.
   b. Have the patient use a sturdy stepstool when the bed is high and not adjustable.
   c. Use tub and shower stools and sturdy handrails in bathrooms.
   d. Have patients in wheelchairs use wide doorways, ramps, and elevators so that they are not tempted to try to walk stairways.
3. The risk factors for accidental falls are (refer to page 379):
   a. Advancing age
   b. Impaired mobility
   c. Confusion
   d. Diarrhea or urinary frequency
   e. Impaired vision
   f. Sedating medications
   g. Postural hypotension
   h. Weakened state
4. When a fire occurs, the nurse should (refer to page 375):
   a. Evacuate the people in the room with the fire.
   b. Close the door to the room with the fire.
   c. Notify the switchboard using the proper code and location for the fire. Do not hang up until the operator repeats the information.
   d. Close all patient room doors and fire doors.
   e. Turn off oxygen in the vicinity of the fire. Use a manual resuscitation mask for patients who need continuous ventilation.
   f. Place moist towels or bath blankets at the threshold of doors where smoke is leaking.
   g. Use the appropriate fire extinguisher if it is a minor fire.
5. When using a fire extinguisher, the nurse should (refer to pages 375–376):
   a. Free the extinguisher from its enclosure.
   b. Remove the pin that locks the handle.
   c. Aim the nozzle near the edge—not the center—of the fire.
   d. Move the nozzle side to side.
   e. Avoid skin contact with the contents of the fire extinguisher.
   f. Return the extinguisher to the maintenance department for replacement or refilling.

CHAPTER 19

Pain Management

The number in parentheses following each rationale indicates on which page in *Fundamental Skills and Concepts in Patient Care*, Seventh Edition, you can find the correct answer.

ANSWERS TO MATCHING QUESTIONS

Items 1 Through 5

(Refer to Display 19-3, page 397)

1. (c)
2. (d)
3. (b)
4. (e)
5. (a)
6. (f)
7. (c)
8. (g)
9. (d)
10. (a)

Items 6 Through 10

(Refer to page 393)

6. (e)
7. (c)
8. (a)
9. (b)
10. (d)

ANSWERS TO MULTIPLE CHOICE QUESTIONS

Items 1 Through 10

1. (b) Pain perception occurs when the pain threshold is reached. Passing the pain threshold results in awareness of discomfort. Pain thresholds tend to be the same among healthy people, but individuals tolerate pain differently. Pain tolerance is influenced by learned behaviors specific to gender, age, and culture. (392)

2. (a) *Acute pain* is physical discomfort of short duration. Short duration is defined as existing less than six months; for most, it is shorter than this. *Chronic pain* is physical discomfort that usually lasts longer than six months. (393–394)

3. (d) *Referred pain* is pain perceived in another location some distance from the body part that is diseased or injured. For example, although heart pain is usually felt in the chest, it may be felt in the arms, neck, and even jaw. (393)

4. (b) The exact nature in which acupuncture and acupressure work has not been definitely determined. The gate-control theory is used by some to explain their effectiveness. Others believe that acupuncture and acupressure may stimulate the body's production of endogenous opioids, chemicals produced by the body that have pain-relieving qualities. (405)

5. (c) *Biofeedback* consists of a training program that helps a person become aware of certain body changes. The individual then learns to alter these physical responses. (408–409)

6. (d) A placebo is an inactive substance given as a substitute for drug therapy. Studies have shown that placebos can be effective pain relievers when not used on a continuous basis and when the patient has confidence in his health caretakers. It is wrong to assume that a patient relieved of pain with placebos is a malingerer or is imagining his pain. (411)

7. (c) TENS has several advantages. It is a nonnarcotic, noninvasive agent without toxic effects. It is contraindicated for pregnant individuals because its effect on the unborn has not been determined. (405)

8. (b) The equianalgesic dose would be morphine sulfate 30 mg by mouth every 3 to 4 hours. (See Table 19-4, page 410)

9. (d) The term *equianalgesic* dose of a medication refers to the adjusted oral dose of the medication that provides the same level of relief as the parenteral dose. (410)

10. (b) Nondrug interventions are most likely to be used for patients with chronic pain or for those patients for whom acute pain management techniques are unsuccessful or contraindicated. (404)

ANSWERS TO TRUE OR FALSE QUESTIONS

Items 1 Through 12

1. *False.* Pain threshold is the point at which the sensation of pain becomes noticeable. *Pain tolerance* is the ability of the individual to endure pain. (392)

2. *False.* Phantom limb pain is pain that is felt in a missing arm or leg. Discomfort in a location distant from the diseased or injured part of the body is known as *referred pain.* (393)

3. *True.*

4. *False.* Pain has cultural implications. In some cultures, people learn to bear pain bravely and behave as though it is hardly present, even when it is severe. However, a person from another culture may learn to express emotions and to show great concern and anxiety about pain. (392)

5. *True.*

6. *False.* The body does not adapt to pain as it does to heat, cold, noise, and odors. (391–394)

7. *True.*

8. *False.* Patient-controlled analgesia infusers are used in hospitals primarily to relieve acute pain following surgery. (398)

9. *False.* The initial dose is slightly higher to establish an acceptable serum level of the drug and provide reduction in pain. (399)

10. *True.*

11. *True.*

12. *True.*

ANSWER TO SHORT ANSWER QUESTIONS

Items 1 Through 2.

1. The advantages to both the patient and the nurse when a patient controlled analgesia is used are (refer to page 399):
   a. Pain relief is rapidly experienced because the drug is delivered directly into the bloodstream.
   b. Pain is maintained within a constant tolerable level.
   c. Less total narcotic is actually used because the discomfort rarely falls below a tolerable range.
   d. The patient avoids the additional discomfort of multiple injections into muscle or subcutaneous tissue.
   e. Anxiety is reduced since the patient's pain does not intensify while the patient waits for the nurse to administer medication.
   f. Extremes in drug side effects, such as sedation and respiratory depression, are avoided with lower doses.
   g. Complications associated with immobility, such as blood clots and pneumonia, are reduced because the patient ambulates or moves about more.
   h. The patient takes an active role in his treatment.
   i. The patient's sense of control and independence is preserved.
   j. Use of a PCA infuser frees the nurse to provide other adjunctive pain-relieving measures.

2. Five components of pain assessment are (refer to Table 19-2, page 395):
   a. Onset—time or circumstances under which pain became apparent
   b. Quality—degree of suffering
   c. Intensity—the magnitude of the pain
   d. Location—the anatomical site
   e. Duration—time span of pain

CHAPTER 20

Oxygenation

The number in parentheses following each rationale indicates on which page in *Fundamental Skills and Concepts in Patient Care,* Seventh Edition, you can find the correct answer.

ANSWERS TO MATCHING QUESTIONS

Items 1 Through 10

(Refer to Chapter 20 text)

1. (d)
2. (e)
3. (h)
4. (a)
5. (j)

Items 11 Through 14

(Refer to pages 427–430)

11. (d)
12. (c)
13. (a)
14. (b)

ANSWERS TO MULTIPLE CHOICE QUESTIONS

Items 1 Through 10

1. (a) The patient's responses to oxygen therapy are most accurately determined by pulse oximetry. Observations of the patient are also important for judging responses prior to and concurrent with oxygen therapy. (416)
2. (b) Oxygen becomes progressively toxic at high concentrations. Signs of oxygen toxicity include a dry cough, which may eventually become moist as lung damage occurs, chest pain felt beneath the sternum, nasal stuffiness, nausea and vomiting, and restlessness. (Display 20–2, page 437)
3. (d) An oxygen tank should be cracked before the humidifier and gauge are attached. To *crack* a tank means to briefly open the valve and release oxygen to clear the outlet of dust and other debris. (424)
4. (a) If the patient has a chronic lung ailment, 2 to 3 liters per minute are prescribed. (427)
5. (c) For a patient with a chronic lung condition, high levels of oxygen may decrease or even stop respirations because his body is accustomed to higher than normal carbon dioxide levels. If the chronically high carbon dioxide level falls too low, it no longer acts as one of the normal stimulants of respirations. (427)
6. (d) The Venturi mask allows air to enter the mask and exhaled carbon dioxide to leave the mask at special ports. It can supply up to 40% oxygen. (Table 20–4, page 429)
7. (a) The lung collapses due to the loss of negative pressure within the pleural space. The atmospheric air, which is higher in pressure, moves into and remains within the pleural space. The lung is no longer able to completely expand during each inhalation. (437)
8. (d) The water-seal drainage system is designed to prevent atmospheric air from reentering the pleural space by partially filling one of the chambers in the drainage device with water. As the air and blood drain from the pleural space via the catheters, the lung will gradually reexpand. (437)
9. (b) Because oxygen is being delivered constantly to the lower airway, patients with transtracheal oxygen usually achieve adequate oxygenation with lower liter flows. (436)
10. (c) Oxygen is drying to the mucous membranes. Therefore, oxygen is humidified, in most cases, when 4L/min is administered for an extended period of time. (426)

ANSWERS TO TRUE OR FALSE QUESTIONS

Items 1 Through 10

1. *False. Hypoxia* is defined as a deficiency in the amount of oxygen in inspired air; it is also a term that has come to mean a condition in which cells and tissues are receiving an inadequate supply of oxygen. *Hypoxemia* is a condition in which there is a less than adequate level of oxygen in the blood.   (416)
2. *False.* Oxygen supports combustion but is not flammable.   (436)
3. *False.* A nonrebreathing mask, which provides the patient with the highest concentration of oxygen, is most often used for persons suffering with smoke inhalation or carbon monoxide poisoning.   (427)
4. *False.* Lung collapse is due to the loss of negative pressure within the pleural space. The atmospheric air, which is higher in pressure, moves into and remains within the pleural space, and the lung can no longer completely expand during each inhalation.   (437)
5. *True.*
6. *False.* Do not empty the water-seal drainage collection container routinely. Emptying the collection chamber increases the risk that air will enter the pleural space when the equipment is disconnected.   (Skill 20-3, page 442)
7. *True.*
8. *False.* A nasal cannula's advantage is that it does not interfere with eating, drinking, or talking.   (428)
9. *False.* The respiratory center of patients with chronic pulmonary diseases adapt to elevated levels of carbon dioxide in the blood. The stimulus to breathe comes from sensing a low level of oxygen. If high percentages of oxygen are administered to chronic lung disease patients, respirations slow and the patient may even stop breathing.   (427)
10. *True.*

ANSWERS TO SHORT ANSWER QUESTIONS

Items 1 Through 5
1. Nursing guidelines for the safe use of oxygen are (refer to page 437):
   a. Post "Oxygen in Use" signs whenever oxygen is stored or in use.
   b. Prohibit the burning of candles during religious rites.
   c. Check that electrical devices have a three-pronged plug.
   d. Inspect electrical equipment for the presence of frayed wires or loose connections.
   e. Avoid petroleum products, aerosol products like hair spray, and products containing acetone like nail polish remover where oxygen is used.
   f. Secure portable cylinders to rigid stands.
2. Common signs of inadequate oxygenation are (refer to Display 20-1, page 417):
   a. Restlessness
   b. Rapid, shallow breathing
   c. Rapid heart rate
   d. Sitting up to breathe
   e. Nasal flaring
   f. Use of accessory muscles
   g. Hypertension
   h. Confusion, stupor, coma
   i. Cyanosis of the skin, lips, and nailbeds
3. Evaluation components are (refer to Skill 20-2, pages 434–435):
   a. Respiratory rate is 12 to 24 breaths per minute at rest.
   b. Breathing is effortless.
   c. Heart rate is <100 bpm.
   d. Patient is alert and oriented.
   e. Skin and mucous membranes are normal color.
   f. SaO_2 is $\geq$ 90%.
   g. FIO_2 and delivery device correspond to medical order.
4. Actions taken when administering oxygen from a tank include (refer to pages 424–427):
   a. Be sure the tank contains oxygen and not some other gas.
   b. Crack the tank to remove dust and debris before attaching the gauges.
   c. Attach a humidifier to the tank and fill it with water.
   d. Stabilize the tank at the bedside on a rigid standard with belts.
5. Methods of administering oxygen include (refer to pages 427–436):
   a. Nasal catheter
   b. Nasal cannula
   c. Various masks
   d. Tent
   e. Into a tracheostomy

CHAPTER 21

Asepsis

The number in parentheses following each rationale indicates on which page in *Fundamental Skills and Concepts in Patient Care*, Seventh Edition, you can find the correct answer.

ANSWERS TO MATCHING QUESTIONS

Items 1 through 5

(Refer to Table 21-1, page 452)

1. (c)	6. (g)
2. (e)	7. (c)
3. (b)	8. (i)
4. (a)	9. (f)
5. (d)	10. (b)

Items 6 through 10

(Refer to pages 450–451)

6. (d)	
7. (b)	
8. (e)	
9. (a)	
10. (c)	

ANSWERS TO MULTIPLE CHOICE QUESTIONS

Items 1 Through 16

1. (a)   Microorganisms, or what most people call germs, are everywhere, but they cannot be seen without a microscope. Many are harmless; they are called *nonpathogens*. Those which cause infections or contagious diseases are called *pathogens*.   (450)

2. (c)   Following generations of reproduction, many microorganisms have gradually changed. One example of an adaptive change is the ability to become spore-forming.   (451)

3. (d)   The port of entry is the part of the body where organisms enter. Examples include any break in the skin or mucous membranes, mouth, nose, and genitourinary tract.   (453)

4. (b)   The vehicle of transmission is the means by which organisms are carried about. Examples include hands, equipment (e.g., bedpan), instruments, china and silverware, linen, and droplets. (Table 21-1, page 452)

5. (b)   Soaps and detergents can be considered antimicrobial agents. An antimicrobial agent is a chemical that kills or suppresses the growth or reproduction of microorganisms.   (Table 21-2, page 454)

6. (a)   *Antiseptics* are chemical agents used to reduce the growth of microorganisms on living tissue. This category of anti-infective agents only prevents or inhibits the growth and reproduction of microorganisms. They do not completely destroy all microbes; therefore, their use is not a form of sterilization.   (454)

7. (c)   A *disinfectant* is a bacteriocidal substance. A bacteriocide is a substance that is capable of destroying or killing microorganisms, but not necessarily spores. These antimicrobials are not intended for use on people.   (454)

8. (d)   Nosocomial infections are infections acquired after being admitted to a health care agency.   (453)

9. (d)   Handwashing is the most frequently used medical aseptic practice in health care agencies. It is the most effective way to prevent nosocomial infections.   (453 and 455)

10. (b)   The care given to cleaning contaminated supplies and equipment throughout the time a person is a patient in a health care agency is called *concurrent disinfection*. When the patient is discharged, all the contaminated supplies and equipment are cleaned a final time in order to get them ready for use by another patient. This is called *terminal disinfection*.   (463)

303

11. (c) Dry heat, or hot-air sterilization, uses equipment similar to a home baking oven. It is a good way to sterilize sharp instruments and reusable syringes because moist heat damages cutting edges and the ground surfaces of glass. (464)

12. (c) Surgical asepsis is based on the underlying principle that equipment and areas that are free of microorganisms must be protected from contamination. (465)

13. (a) A sterile field is a work area that is free of microorganisms. The inner surface of a wrapper that holds sterilized equipment is often used as a sterile field much like a tablecloth would be used. The nurse must open the sterile package in such a way as to keep the inside of the wrapper and its contents sterile. This may be done by positioning the wrapped package so that the outermost triangular edge can be moved away from the nurse when the sealed tape is broken or removed. (465)

14. (c) A sterile package should be opened by unfolding the wrapper on the far side of the package first and the nearest side last. The risk of contamination is increased by reaching over a sterile area. (465)

15. (b) Opened wrappers are considered sterile within 1 inch of the edge. The sterile margin of a peeled package is its inner edge. (465)

16. (b) Talking, coughing, and sneezing over a sterile area must be avoided. Microorganisms are present in the moisture from respiratory secretions. These droplets can fall onto sterile areas causing contamination. (459–461)

ANSWERS TO TRUE OR FALSE QUESTIONS

Items 1 Through 10

1. *False.* A microbe that requires free oxygen in order to exist is called an *aerobic microorganism.* Anerobic microorganisms depend on an environment without oxygen for survival. (450)
2. *True.*
3. *True.*
4. *False.* The *reservoir* is a place on which or in which microorganisms grow and reproduce. A person or animal on which or in which microorganisms live is called the *host.* (453)
5. *False.* Medical asepsis (clean technique) refers to the practices that help confine or reduce the number of microorganisms, especially pathogens. (453)
6. *False.* Handwashing is the single most effective way to prevent nosocomial infections. (455)

7. *False.* Antibiotics have saved many patients' lives. However, they are only useful in reducing or destroying the growth of bacteria, one type of microorganism. Even so, not *all* bacteria are affected by all antibiotics. (454)
8. *False.* Rinse items first under *cool,* running water. Hot water causes many substances to coagulate (that is to thicken or congeal), making them difficult to remove. (463)
9. *True.*
10. *False.* Objects may be soaked in a 70% solution for 10 to 20 minutes. This is *not* considered a reliable sterilization method; its action should be regarded more as that of an antimicroabial agent. (454)

ANSWERS TO SHORT ANSWER QUESTIONS

Items 1 Through 5

1. The conditions most microorganisms need to grow and survive are (refer to page 451):
   a. Warmth
   b. Air
   c. Water
   d. Darkness
   e. Nourishment
2. The factors that can result in reduced resistance to the entry of disease-causing organisms are (refer to Display 21-2, page 453):
   a. Poor nutrition
   b. Poor personal hygiene
   c. Broken skin or mucous membranes
   d. Aging
   e. Illness
   f. Suppressed immune system
3. The guidelines for safe and effective practices of medical asepsis when soap or detergents and water are used to clean supplies and equipment are (refer to page 463):
   a. Wear waterproof gloves if items are heavily contaminated.
   b. Disassemble equipment immediately after use.
   c. Rinse items first under cool, running water.
   d. Rinse catheters and rectal tubes immediately after use to remove lubricant or body excretions.
   e. Use water and soap or detergent for cleaning purposes.
   f. Use a brush with stiff bristles to loosen dirt as necessary.
   g. Force sudsy water through the openings of reusable needles and other hollow channels.

h. Rinse items well under running water after cleaning with soap or detergent and water.
i. Air dry equipment.
j. Treat gloves, brushes, sponges, cleaning cloths, and water used for cleaning as reservoirs for microorganisms.
k. Avoid splashing or spilling water on yourself or on the floor or other equipment during the entire procedure.
l. Consider hands heavily contaminated after cleaning equipment. Even when wearing gloves during cleaning, handwashing should be performed.

4. The body is capable of producing additional specialized cells and chemicals that are responsible for inhibiting the growth and spread of microorganisms. (453)

5. Handwashing should be performed (refer to Display 21-3, page 459):
a. When arriving and leaving work
b. Before and after contact with each patient
c. Before and after equipment is handled
d. Before and after gloving
e. Before and after specimens are collected
f. Before preparing medications
g. Before serving trays or feeding patients
h. Before eating
i. After toileting, haircombing, or other hygiene
j. After cleaning a work area

CHAPTER 22

Infection Control

The number in parentheses following each rationale indicates on which page in *Fundamental Skills and Concepts in Patient Care,* Seventh Edition, you can find the correct answer.

ANSWERS TO MATCHING QUESTIONS

Items 1 Through 5

(Refer to Table 22-1, page 476)

1. (d)
2. (e)
3. (a)
4. (c)
5. (b)

ANSWERS TO MULTIPLE CHOICE QUESTIONS

Items 1 Through 10

1. (a)   An *infection* is a condition that results when microorganisms cause injury to their host.   (475)
2. (c)   Infection control refers to physical measures that attempt to curtail the spread of infectious or contagious diseases.   (476)
3. (c)   Handwashing is the single most effective means of preventing the spread of microorganisms. (Refer to chapter 21)
4. (a)   Gloves are required when an infectious disease is transmissible by direct contact or contact with blood or body substances.   (480)
5. (d)   Standard Precautions are infection-control measures to be used when caring for all patients in hospitals regardless of their infectious status. Standard Precautions combine what was previously referred to as Universal Precautions and Body Substance Isolation.   (476)

6. (c)   To control the spread of most communicable diseases in a health agency, the patient is placed in a private room. In this way, no other patient is in direct contact with the infected or susceptible person.   (479)
7. (b)   Rubella is an example of a disease requiring droplet precautions.   (Table 22-2, page 478)
8. (a)   Diarrhea is an example of a disease requiring contact precautions.   (478)
9. (b)   Chickenpox is an example of a disease requiring airborne precautions.   (478)
10. (b)   The current list of body fluids with the potential for containing these infectious viruses includes blood and any body fluid containing visible blood, semen, and vaginal secretions.   (pages 476–477)

ANSWERS TO TRUE OR FALSE QUESTIONS

Items 1 Through 10

1. *False.* In the most recent guidelines from the CDC in 1996, two major categories of infection-control practices were recommended. They are Standard Precautions and Transmission-based Precautions. Standard Precautions combine Universal Precautions and Body Substance Isolation. Transmission-based Precautions replace the previous categories referred to as STRICT Isolation, CONTACT Isolation, RESPIRATORY Isolation, TUBERCULOSIS Isolation, ENTERIC Precautions, and DRAINAGE/SE-CRETION Precautions. The new Transmission-based Precaution categories are Airborne, Droplet, and Contact Precautions.   (476–477)
2. *True.*
3. *True.*
4. *False.* Droplet spread is the physical transfer of microorganisms between material released from the nose and mouth of an infected person when he coughs, sneezes, and talks and a susceptible host.   (477–478)

5. *True.*
6. *True.*
7. *True.*
8. *False.* Gloves are not a total and complete barrier to microorganisms. Leakage occurs approximately 2% of the time. It increases with the stress of their use. (480)
9. *True.*
10. *False.* Hepatitis B is only one of several diseases that can be spread by blood. So regardless of having received the vaccine, whenever there is a possibility for contact with blood or body fluids that can potentially spread bloodborne viruses, gloves should be worn. (Chapter 22 text)

ANSWERS TO SHORT ANSWER QUESTIONS

Items 1 and 2

1. Standard Precautions are (refer to Display 22-2, page 477):
   a. Wear gloves when touching blood, body fluids, secretions, excretions, mucous membranes, and nonintact skin.
   b. Perform handwashing immediately when there is direct contact with blood, body fluids, secretions, excretions, and contaminated items; after removing gloves; and between patient contacts.
   c. Wear a mask and eye protection, or face shield when there is chance of splashes or sprays of blood, body fluids, secretions, and excretions.
   d. Wear a cover gown when there is chance of sprays or splashing clothing with blood, body fluids, secretions, and excretions.
   e. Remove soiled protective items promptly when potential contact with pathogens is no longer present.
   f. Clean and reprocess all equipment before reuse.
   g. Discard all single-use items in appropriate containers.
   h. Handle, transport, and process soiled linen in a manner that prevents contamination of self, others, and the environment.
   i. Prevent injury with used sharp devices by handling appropriately.
   j. Place patients who contaminate the environment and cannot or do not assist with appropriate hygiene or environmental cleanliness in a private room.
2. Methods of contracting AIDS are (refer to Display 22-1, page 476):
   a. Contact with the blood, semen, or vaginal secretions of an HIV-infected person during unprotected vaginal, anal, or oral sexual intercourse
   b. Contact with the blood, semen, or vaginal secretions of an HIV-infected person during medical, dental, and nursing procedures in which these fluids enter through an open cut or splash into a caregiver's eyes or nose
   c. Contact with the blood of an HIV-infected person by sharing needles, receiving a transfusion of contaminated blood or blood cell components, receiving plasma or clotting factors that have not been heat treated, and contaminated ear-piercing or tattooing equipment
   d. Infected pregnant women may transmit the disease to their infants during pregnancy, at birth, and while breast feeding

CHAPTER 23

Body Mechanics, Positioning, and Moving

The number in parentheses following each rationale indicates on which page in *Fundamental Skills and Concepts in Patient Care,* Seventh Edition, you can find the correct answer.

ANSWERS TO MATCHING QUESTIONS

Items 1 Through 5

(Refer to Table 23-3, page 505)

1. (b)
2. (f)
3. (d)
4. (e)
5. (c)

Items 6 Through 11

(Refer to Table 23-2, page 492)

6. (e)
7. (g)
8. (b)
9. (f)
10. (a)
11. (d)

ANSWERS TO MULTIPLE CHOICE QUESTIONS

Items 1 Through 14

1. (c)   Muscle weakness, atelectasis, and contractures are some of the many problems related to the disuse syndrome.   (Table 23-1, page 492)
2. (b)   Footdrop is a type of contracture that results from prolonged plantar flexion, lack of movement of the ankle joint, and shortening of muscles at the back of the calf.   (495)

3. (b)   *Posture* refers to the position of the body or the way in which it is held.   (466)
4. (b)   Keep the feet parallel and about 10 to 20 cm (4 to 8 inches) apart when in a standing position to give the body a wide base of support.   (492)
5. (a)   Body mechanics is the efficient use of the body as a machine. Using good body mechanics is as important for the nurse as it is for others. Basic principles of body mechanics can be applied regardless of the worker or the task.   (493)
6. (c)   Use the longest and strongest muscles to provide the energy needed for a task. It is best to use the long and strong muscles in the arms, legs, and hips whenever possible. Small and less strong muscles will strain and injure quickly if forced to work beyond their ability. One of the most common injuries affects the muscles in the lower part of the back. It is a painful injury and usually slow to heal, but it is preventable when proper body mechanics are used. (Nursing Guidelines for Using Good Body Mechanics, 494)
7. (b)   Push, pull, or roll objects whenever possible, rather than lift them. It takes more effort to lift something against the force of gravity. Use body weight as a lever to assist with pushing or pulling an object. This reduces the strain placed on a group of muscles.   (494)
8. (a)   Stretching and twisting fatigue muscles quickly. When stretching or twisting, balance will be poor as the line of gravity falls outside the body's base of support.   (494)
9. (a)   An inactive patient's position should be changed at least every 2 hours and more frequently if any signs or symptoms of the disuse syndrome have been assessed.   (494)
10. (a)   A turning sheet is a helpful positioning device. The sheet extends from the upper back to the thighs.   (497)

11. (d) Foam acts almost like a layer of subcutaneous tissue. Foam contains channels and cells filled with air. This allows some evaporation of moisture and escape of heat, which reduces the potential for skin breakdown. (504)

12. (c) There are two primary concerns when using the supine position. One concern is pressure on the back of the body where pressure sores commonly develop, especially in the area at the end of the spine. The second is toe pressure from linens, which, when combined with gravity, forces the feet into the footdrop position. (495)

13. (b) The primary concern when using the lateral position is if the upper shoulder and arm are allowed to rotate forward and fall out of alignment. This tends to interfere with proper breathing. (495)

14. (b) High Fowler's position is especially helpful to patients with dyspnea. It causes abdominal organs to drop away from the diaphragm, relieving pressure on the chest cavity. (496)

ANSWERS TO TRUE OR FALSE QUESTIONS

Items 1 Through 10

1. *False.* Good posture when in the standing position includes holding the head erect with the face forward and with the chin in slightly. (492)

2. *False.* It is important to have good posture when lying down. The muscles are in a state of relaxation when resting or sleeping. Unless the parts of the body are properly supported, the body will respond to gravity and fall out of alignment. Poor alignment makes it difficult for the body to function effectively. (493)

3. *True.*

4. *False.* Egg-crate mattresses provide minimal pressure reduction and are often used for comfort only. Thicker waffle-shaped foams offer greater pressure reduction and can be used for preventing skin breakdown. (504)

5. *False.* Trochanter rolls are placed along the outside of the patient's thighs at the trochanter region of the femur to prevent outward rotation of the legs. (497)

6. *True.*

7. *False.* When transferring a patient from the bed to the chair, the nurse should place the chair alongside the bed on the patient's stronger side. (Skill 23-2, page 509)

8. *True.*

9. *True.*

10. *True.*

ANSWERS TO SHORT ANSWER QUESTIONS

Items 1 Through 5

1. Characteristics of good posture are (refer to Key Concepts, page 515):
   a. Standing:
      1. Keep the feet parallel.
      2. Distribute weight equally on both feet to provide a broad base of support.
   b. Sitting:
      1. The buttocks and upper thighs are the base of support.
      2. Both feet rest on the floor.
   c. Lying:
      1. Looks same as standing but in horizontal position.
      2. Body parts in neutral position.

2. Principles of correct body mechanics are (refer to Key Concepts, page 515):
   a. Distribute gravity through the center of body over a wide base of support.
   b. Push, pull or roll objects rather than lift them.
   c. Hold objects close to the body.

3. Five positioning devices and the purpose of each are (refer to Key Concepts, page 516):
   a. Adjustable bed—Allows the position of the head and knees to be changed.
   b. Pillows—Provide support and elevate body part.
   c. Trochanter rolls—Prevent legs from turning outward.
   d. Hand rolls—Maintain functional use of the hand and prevent contractures.
   e. Foot boards—Keep the feet in normal walking position.

4. Three pressure-relieving devices and an advantage of each are (refer to Key Concepts, page 516):
   a. Siderails—Aid patients in changing their own positions.
   b. Mattress overlays—Reduce pressure and restore skin integrity.
   c. Cradle—Keeps linen off patient's feet or legs.

5. Five measures to prevent inactivity in older adults are (refer to Patient Teaching For Promoting Activity and Mobility, page 514):
   a. Balance periods of activity with periods of rest.
   b. Allow adequate time for performing activities.
   c. Develop hobbies or recreational interests.
   d. Investigate local support groups.
   e. Prevent injury by removing any objects that pose a safety hazard.

CHAPTER 24

Therapeutic Exercise

The number in parentheses following each rationale indicates on which page in *Fundamental Skills and Concepts in Patient Care,* Seventh Edition, you can find the correct answer.

ANSWERS TO MATCHING QUESTIONS

Items 1 Through 11

(Refer to Table 24-4, page 522)

1. (f)
2. (l)
3. (i)
4. (c)
5. (k)
6. (j)
7. (b)
8. (e)
9. (a)
10. (g)
11. (d)

ANSWERS TO MULTIPLE CHOICE QUESTIONS

Items 1 Through 10

1. (c) Exercise is the movement intended to increase strength, stamina, and overall body tone. (517)
2. (a) The preferred type of exercise is *active exercise.* People who are ill may need the assistance of another to move. This type of exercise is known as *passive exercise.* (521)

3. (c) *Isometric exercises* involve contracting and relaxing muscle groups with little, if any, movement. These exercises increase the mass and definition of skeletal muscles, but they do not increase the capacity of the heart and lungs to perform. (521)
4. (c) The formula for computing the target heart rate is: 220 – age × 60% = target heart rate. (520)
5. (a) *Isotonic exercise* is that which involves movement and work. One of the best examples is aerobic exercise. *Aerobic exercise* involves rhythmically moving all parts of the body at a moderate to slow speed without impeding the ability to breathe.
6. (c) Isometric exercise refers to stationary exercises that tend to be performed against a resistive force. (494)
7. (c) The nursing diagnosis "Unilateral Neglect" is defined by NANDA as a state in which an individual is perceptually unaware of and inattentive to one side of the body. (512)
8. (b) A submaximal fitness test is an exercise test that does not stress a person to exhaustion. (518)
9. (c) The term body composition refers to the amount of body tissue that is lean versus that which is fat. (518)
10. (d) Range-of-motion exercises are therapeutic activity in which joints are moved in the positions that the joint normally permits. (521–522).

ANSWERS TO TRUE OR FALSE QUESTIONS

Items 1 Through 15

1. *True.*
2. *True.*
3. *True.*
4. *True.*

5. *False.* Athletes generally have low pulse rates but their cells are adequately oxygenated. Any muscle that is exercised increases in tone. Therefore, because the heart is a muscle, exercise increases its tone and it will be able to pump more blood with less effort. (520)

6. *False.* The amount of movement that is possible in a joint is known as *range of motion*. The range that is available in each joint is referred to as its flexibility. (521–522)

7. *False.* One of the chief minerals that allows bones to be strong and compact is calcium. (Chapter 14)

8. *True.*

9. *True.*

10. *False.* A stress electrocardiogram is done during exercise and records the activity of the heart while the patient walks on a treadmill that moves at a progressively faster pace. (518)

11. *True.*

12. *True.*

13. *False.* According to the National Strategies for Improving Physical Fitness, children should be involved in activities that may be readily carried into adulthood. (Table 24-5, page 533)

14. *True.*

15. *True.*

ANSWERS TO SHORT ANSWER QUESTIONS

Items 1 Through 4

1. Guidelines for assisting with range-of-motion exercises are (refer to Nursing Guidelines for Performing Range-of-Motion Exercises, page 522):
   a. Use good body mechanics.
   b. Remove pillows and other positioning devices.
   c. Position the patient to facilitate moving a joint through all of its usual positions.
   d. Follow a pattern; for example, begin at the head and move toward the feet.
   e. Perform similar movements with each extremity.
   f. Support the joint being exercised.
   g. Move each joint until there is resistance but not pain.
   h. Watch for nonverbal communication.
   i. Avoid exercising a painful joint.
   j. Stop if spasticity develops.
   k. Apply gentle pressure to the muscle or move the joint more slowly.
   l. Expect that the patient's vital signs will increase during exercise but return to resting rate.
   m. Teach the family to perform range of motion with the patient.

2. Five benefits of physical exercise are (refer to Display 24-1, page 518):
   a. Improved cardiopulmonary function
   b. Reduction of blood pressure
   c. Increased muscle tone and strength
   d. Greater physical endurance
   e. Increased lean mass and weight loss
   f. Reduction of elevated blood sugar
   g. Decreased low-density blood lipids
   h. Improved physical appearance
   i. Increased bone density
   j. Regularity of bowel elimination
   k. Promotion of sleep
   l. Reduction in tension and depression

3. Four national strategies for improving physical activity and fitness are (refer to Table 24-5, page 533):
   a. Increase daily participation in physical education in elementary and secondary schools.
   b. Include more physical activity during physical education classes.
   c. Involve children in physical activities that may be readily carried into adulthood.
   d. Increase employer-sponsored physical activities and fitness programs.
   e. Increase community availability and accessibility to physical activity and fitness facilities.
   f. Increase counseling and the provision of exercise prescriptions for patients under the care of a physician.

4. Items necessary for patient teaching in order to develop a safe exercise program are (refer to Patient Teaching for a Safe Exercise Program, page 521):
   a. Seek a pre-exercise fitness evaluation.
   b. Identify activities within one's prescribed level of METs.
   c. Choose a form of exercise that seems pleasurable and involves as many muscle groups as possible.
   d. Plan three days of exercise per week at a convenient time of day.
   e. Exercise with a partner for safety and motivational purposes.
   f. Avoid exercising in extreme weather conditions, such as when there is high humidity or when smog is evident.
   g. Dress in layers according to the temperature and weather conditions.
   h. Purchase supportive footwear.

i. Wear reflective clothing when on the roadside.

j. Walk or jog against traffic; cycle in the same direction as traffic.

k. Eat complex carbohydrates (pasta, rice, cooked cereal) rather than fasting or eating simple sugars (cookies, chocolate, sweetened drinks).

l. Avoid drinking alcohol, which dilates the blood vessels, promotes heat loss, and interferes with good judgment.

m. Calculate one's target heart rate (maximum heart rate × 60%).

n. Warm up for five minutes by stretching muscle groups or doing light calisthenics.

o. Monitor heart rate two or three times while exercising.

p. Slow the pace down if the heart rate exceeds one's pre-established target.

q. Try to sustain the target heart rate for at least 20 minutes.

r. Never stop exercising abruptly.

s. Cool down for at least five minutes in a manner similar to one's warm-up.

CHAPTER 25

Mechanical Immobilization

The number in parentheses following each rationale indicates on which page in *Fundamental Skills and Concepts in Patient Care,* Seventh Edition, you can find the correct answer.

ANSWERS TO MATCHING QUESTIONS

Items 1 through 6

(Refer to Chapter 25 text.)

1. (c)
2. (e)
3. (f)
4. (b)
5. (a)
6. (d)

ANSWERS TO MULTIPLE CHOICE QUESTIONS

Items 1 Through 10

1. (d)   Orthoses are orthopedic devices that support or align a body part and prevent or correct deformities.   (537)
2. (c)   A cervical collar is a foam or rigid splint around the neck. It is used to treat athletic neck injuries or other trauma that results in a neck strain or sprain.   (539)
3. (c)   Apply the splinting device so that it spans the injured area from the joint above the injury to beyond the joint below the injury. For instance, if the lower leg has been injured, the splint should be long enough to restrict movement of the knee and ankle.   (538)
4. (c)   A triangular sling used to support the arm is applied as follows:

- Place the open triangle on the patient's chest with the base of the triangle along the length of the patient's chest on the unaffected side.
- Place the upper end of the base of the triangle around the back of the neck on the unaffected side.
- Place the apex or point of the triangle under the affected arm.
- Place the lower end of the base of the triangle across the affected arm.
- Tie the two ends of the base of a triangle in a knot at the side of the neck.
- Be sure the hand is higher than the elbow in the sling to prevent swelling in the hand.
- Fold and secure the material on the affected side neatly. A pin may be used, behind the sling so that it is out of sight, to secure the material.   (542)

5. (a)   Plaster casts may remain wet for 24 to 48 hours, depending on the level of humidity in the air.   (Table 25-1, page 545)
6. (d)   Ordinarily, the air circulation in the room is adequate for drying the layers of plaster.   (546)
7. (b)   Because most casts are applied after an injury and surgical procedure, the nurse may expect that the area will swell and bleed. The extent of swelling and bleeding are the two immediate problems with which the nurse must be concerned. Swelling is especially serious since the cast is rigid and will not expand as the area within the cast becomes larger. The cast can create a tourniquet effect.   (546)
8. (c)   One assessment technique for determining the extent and effects of swelling and circulation involves performing the blanching test. Swelling affects blood flow. The nurse compares the data on the appearance and sensation in the fingernails or toes to determine if circulation is impaired. A radial or pedal pulse may or may not be palpated, depending on the length of the cast.   (546 & 548)

9. (c)   Examination and treatment should take place within 30–45 minutes after a pneumatic splint has been applied, or circulation may be affected.   (531)

10. (a)   Braces are custom-made devices designed to support weakened structures during periods of activity.   (541)

ANSWERS TO TRUE OR FALSE QUESTIONS

Items 1 Through 12

1. *False.* A *brace* is designed to support weakened body structures during weight bearing. A *splint* is a device that immobilizes and protects an injured part of the body.   (538 & 541)

2. *True.*

3. *False.* Inflate a pneumatic splint to the point that it can be indented only 1.3 cm (1/2 inch) with the fingertips.   (539)

4. *False.* Casts made of the newer synthetic materials dry quickly. These casts become rigid so quickly that the patient may bear weight within 15 to 30 minutes of application. On the other hand, plaster casts may remain wet for 24 to 48 hours, depending on the level of humidity in the air.   (Table 25-1, page 545)

5. *True.*

6. *False.* Expose the cast directly to the air. A cast produces heat as it dries. If the cast is covered, moisture accumulates and evaporation is delayed.   (546)

7. *False.* The blanching test is done to determine the extent and effects of swelling and circulation.   (546)

8. *False.* Venous and capillary bleeding under a cast are characterized by a reddish-brown stain on the cast.

9. *True.*

10. *False.* The physician usually uses an electric cast cutter to separate and remove the cast. A cast cutter is a noisy instrument that can be frightening to a patient. There is a natural expectation that an instrument sharp enough to cut a cast would be sharp enough to lacerate several layers of tissue. However, when used properly, an electric cast cutter should leave the skin intact.   (549)

11. *False.* After the removal of a cast, the skin may be washed as usual with soapy warm water but the semi-attached areas of loose skin should not be forcibly removed. Lotion applied to the skin may add moisture and prevent rough edges from catching on clothing.   (549)

12. *False.* For patients in skeletal traction, active range of motion along with isometric and isotonic exercise should be encouraged. Body areas that are unrestricted by traction should be kept flexible and in good tone. Isometric exercises may be performed on the areas where motion is restricted.   (552)

ANSWERS TO SHORT ANSWER QUESTIONS

Items 1 Through 4

1. General purposes of mechanical immobilization are to (refer to page 538):
   a. Relieve pain and muscle spasm.
   b. Support and align damaged tissues.
   c. Restrict movement while injuries heal.
   d. Maintain functional positions until healing is complete.
   e. Allow activity while restricting movement of an injured area.
   f. Prevent further structural damage and deformity.

2. Important techniques that should be followed when applying an emergency splint are (refer to Nursing Guidelines for Applying an Emergency Splint, page 538):
   a. Avoid changing the position of an injured part of the body even if it appears grossly deformed.
   b. Leave a high-top shoe or a ski boot in place if an injured ankle is suspected.
   c. Select a splint or substitute splint material that will not permit movement of the body part once it is applied.
   d. Apply the splinting device so that it spans the injured area from the joint above the injury to beyond the joint below the injury.
   e. Inflate a pneumatic splint to the point that it can be indented only 1.3 centimeters (1/2 inch) with the fingertips. Avoid inflation longer than 30 to 45 minutes or circulation in the area may be affected.
   f. Use an uninjured area of the body adjacent to the injured part if no other sturdy material is available.
   g. Cover any open wounds with clean material to absorb blood and prevent the entrance of dirt and additional pathogens.
   h. Apply soft material over any area of the body that may be subject to pressure or rubbing by areas on an inflexible splint.

i. Use tape or wide strips of fabric in several areas to confine the injured part to the splint so that it cannot be moved. Narrow cord can create a tourniquet effect, especially if it encircles swelling tissue.

j. Assess the color and temperature of fingers or toes to evaluate if blood flow is adequate. Loosen the attached device if the fingers or toes appear pale, blue, or cold.

k. Elevate the entire length of the immobilized part so that the lowest point is higher than the heart.

l. Provide for the individual's warmth and safety and seek assistance in transporting the injured person to a health agency.

3. Types of casts are (refer to page 541):
   a. Cylinder casts
   b. Body casts
   c. Spica casts

4. Principles for maintaining effective traction are (refer to Display 25-1, page 552):
   a. Traction must produce a pulling effect on the body.
   b. Countertraction (counterpull) must be maintained.
   c. The pull of traction and the counterpull must be in exactly opposite directions.
   d. Splints and slings must be suspended without interference.
   e. Ropes must move freely through each pulley.
   f. The prescribed amount of weight must be applied.
   g. The weights must hang free.

CHAPTER 26

Ambulatory Aids

The number in parentheses following each rationale indicates on which page in *Fundamental Skills and Concepts in Patient Care*, Seventh Edition, you can find the correct answer.

ANSWERS TO MATCHING QUESTIONS

Items 1 Through 4

(Refer to Table 26-1, page 552)

1. (c)
2. (d)
3. (a)
4. (b)

ANSWERS TO MULTIPLE CHOICE QUESTIONS

Items 1 Through 10

1. (a)   Muscle tone refers to the ability of muscles to respond when stimulated. Strength is the power to perform.   (547)
2. (c)   Quadriceps setting, sometimes shortened to quad setting, is a form of isometric exercise in which the quadriceps group of muscles are alternately tensed and relaxed.   (548)
3. (b)   For optimum use, a cane must be adjusted to an appropriate height for the patient. When fitted correctly, the cane's handle is parallel with the patient's hip, which should provide approximately a 15-degree angle of elbow flexion.   (550)
4. (d)   Platform crutches are designed to support the forearm. They are especially useful for patients unable to bear weight with their hands and wrists. Many patients with arthritis use them.   (551)
5. (d)   The most stable form of ambulatory aid is the walker; straight canes are the least stable.   (550)
6. (d)   Quadriceps setting is an isometric exercise in which muscles on the front of the thigh are alternatively tensed and relaxed. The patient contracts the quadriceps femoris muscles by pulling the kneecaps toward his hips. The patient will feel that he is pushing his knee down into the mattress and pulling his foot forward.   (548)
7. (b)   The cane should be placed about 10 cm (4 inches) to the side of the foot. It should be held in the hand on the uninvolved side.   (550)
8. (b)   The individual should use the three-point gait for crutch walking when weight bearing is allowed on one leg. The other foot cannot bear weight or can only bear limited weight.   (552)
9. (c)   When using a cane on stairs use the stair rail rather than the cane to go up or down. Take each step up with the stronger leg, followed by the weaker one. Reverse the pattern for descending the stairs. If there is no stair rail, advance the cane just before rising or descending with the weaker leg. (Refer to Patient Teaching for Using a Cane, page 550)
10. (a)   When using a walker, patients are instructed to stand within the walker.   (551)

ANSWERS TO TRUE OR FALSE QUESTIONS

Items 1 Through 10

1. *True.*
2. *True.*
3. *False.* There should be room for two fingers in the space between the top of the axillary bar of the crutch and the fold of the axilla when the patient stands. This prevents injury to the tissues and the nerves in the axilla.   (556)
4. *True.*
5. *False.* The nurse should hold on to the handles of the walking belt and walk alongside the patient.   (550)
6. *True.*

316

7. *True.*

8. *False.* When walking downstairs while using a cane, take each step with the weaker leg first followed by the stronger one. The reverse is true when going up the stairs.   (550)

9. *True.*

10. *False.* Just before the patient is placed on a tilt table, the nurse applies elastic stockings. These stockings help to compress vein walls, thus preventing pooling of blood in the extremities which may trigger fainting.   (549)

ANSWERS TO SHORT ANSWER QUESTIONS

Items 1 Through 4

1. Devices and techniques that provide support and assistance with walking are (refer to page 549):
   a. Parallel bars
   b. Stable pieces of furniture
   c. Walking belts
   d. The nurse

2. Three common aids for ambulation are (refer to page 550):
   a. Cane
   b. Walker
   c. Crutches

3. Three characteristics of appropriately fitted crutches are (refer to page 550):
   a. They permit the patient to stand upright with shoulders relaxed.
   b. They provide space for two fingers between the axilla and the axillary bar.
   c. They facilitate approximately 30 degrees of elbow flexion and slight hyperextension of the wrist.

4. The tilt table is used to help patients get acclimatized to being upright and bearing weight on their own feet.   (549)

CHAPTER 27

Perioperative Care

The number in parentheses following each rationale indicates on which page in *Fundamental Skills and Concepts in Patient Care,* Seventh Edition, you can find the correct answer.

ANSWERS TO MATCHING QUESTIONS

Items 1 Through 5

(Refer to Table 27-1, page 570)

1. (d)
2. (c)
3. (a)
4. (e)
5. (b)

Items 6 Through 12

(Refer to Table 27-5, page 578)

6. (c)
7. (g)
8. (f)
9. (a)
10. (d)
11. (e)
12. (h)

ANSWERS TO MULTIPLE CHOICE QUESTIONS

Items 1 Through 10

1. (d) The primary disadvantage of outpatient surgery is that it reduces the time for establishing a nurse-patient relationship. Since the patient does not come into the hospital until the morning of surgery, there is often very little time for the nurses to work with her prior to the time of the operative procedure.   (Table 27-3, page 571)

2. (b) Regional anesthesia produces loss of feeling in a large area of the body, such as the pelvis and lower extremities, by instilling an anesthetic agent into the spinal canal.   (Table 27-2, page 571)

3. (b) Directed donors must meet all the criteria of a public donor.   (See Table 27-4, page 573)

4. (d) Emotional care continues during the postoperative period in a manner similar to that in preoperative care. The nurse should be alert to feelings and worries that patients may not be able to specifically express. For example, the patient may ask, "How am I doing?" when he really means, "Do you think I'll make it? The nurse may need to interpret the patient's underlying question and explain what is happening to the extent to which individuals are interested or able to understand. (Applicable Nursing Diagnoses, page 579)

5. (c) Deep-breathing and, in some cases, coughing are important measures to prevent the possibility of hypostatic pneumonia and atelectasis.   (573)

6. (b) The patient should be taught forced coughing. Forced coughing is most appropriate for patients who have diminished or moist lung sounds.   (573)

7. (d) Inactivity and gravity cause blood to pool and settle in lower areas of the body. The temporarily inactive surgical patient can perform leg exercises to promote circulation and prevent the formation of blood clots.   (574)

8. (c) Psychological support not only involves providing information, it includes observing and taking the time to listen to the patient and others who are concerned about the patient. It is usually of no help simply to say that everything will be all right and that there is no cause for worry. The helpful nurse will be available to provide an opportunity for individuals to talk about their problems and express feelings. (Review Communication)

318

9. (c)   The smell, nausea, burning, and watering of the eyes, although uncomfortable, are not hazardous. It is the potential inhalation of airborne cells and viruses that is. A conventional mask, even doubled, is not sufficient in filtering substances that measure less than 0.30 micron. Viruses can be as small as 0.12 micron. Thus it is possible, but not proven, that the HIV virus could be transmitted by inhaling the laser plume.   (570)

10. (a)   Assure a child that he will not be left alone. Encourage him to talk about his fears as much as he is able. Tell him it is all right to cry, answer his questions, and correct the misconceptions most children have of surgery. (Review Communication)

ANSWERS TO TRUE OR FALSE QUESTIONS

Items 1 Through 15

1. *False. Evisceration* is the separation of a wound with exposure of body organs. *Dehiscence* is only the separation of a wound. (Table 27-5, page 570)

2. *False.* Patients scheduled for outpatient surgery usually come to the hospital on the day of the operative procedure.   (570)

3. *True.*

4. *True.*

5. *False.* Recent studies have shown controversy about the traditional approach used to prepare the surgical site. This included shaving the body in a wide area surrounding the eventual incision. Shaving is done to remove microorganisms attached to the hair. The theory is valid. However, it has been found that a razor causes microabrasions. When skin is abraded, it allows an entry site for microorganisms. These microbes tend to grow even more vigorously in the plasma-rich environment of the impaired skin. Their growth compounds during the time between shaving and the actual surgery. (575)

6. *False.* The individual who is donating blood as a directed donor must weigh at least 110 pounds.   (550)

7. *False.* The directed donor may donate one unit every 56 days.   (550)

8. *False.* It is generally agreed that, unless moist secretions can be heard in the lungs, forced coughing should not be routinely performed postoperatively.   (557)

9. *True.*

10. *False.* The skin cannot be sterilized, but measures can be taken to reduce the chances of introducing organisms into the operative site.   (552)

11. *True.*

12. *False.* Family members appreciate knowing where they may wait and how long the patient is expected to be in the operating and recovery rooms. It is better not to predict specific times. Delays sometimes occur, causing relatives unnecessary worry.   (576)

13. *False.* When teaching patients deep-breathing exercises, emphasize that the breathing should be done slowly.   (573)

14. *False.* Apply antiembolism stockings in the morning before the patient is out of bed or after elevating the feet for at least 15 minutes. Before the feet are lowered, there is a minimal amount of pooled blood in the lower legs and feet. Elevation helps gravity move blood toward the heart. (Skill 27-1, page 583)

15. *True.*

ANSWERS TO SHORT ANSWER QUESTIONS

Items 1 Through 4

1. The equipment and supplies needed in the postoperative patient's room are (refer to page 577):
    a. Blood pressure equipment
    b. Extra tissue wipes
    c. Emesis basin
    d. I.V. pole

2. The advantages of laser surgery, besides cost-effectiveness, are (refer to page 570):
    a. Reduced need for anesthesia
    b. Smaller incisions
    c. Minimal blood loss
    d. Reduced swelling around the incision
    e. Less pain following the procedure
    f. Decreased incidence of wound infection
    g. Reduced scarring
    h. Less time recuperating

3. Areas commonly addressed in discharge instructions include (refer to page 579):
    a. How to care for the incision site
    b. Signs of complications to report
    c. What drugs to use for relieving pain
    d. How to self-administer prescribed drugs
    e. When presurgical activity can be resumed
    f. If and how much weight can be lifted
    g. Which foods to consume or avoid
    h. When and where to return for a medical appointment.

4. General types of measures included in postoperative orders are (refer to pages 577–579):

   a. The frequency with which vital signs are to be checked once they have stabilized

   b. The type, amount, and rate at which I.V. fluid therapy is to be administered

   c. The concentration and method for administering oxygen

   d. Medications to be given following surgery (ordinarily, orders include drugs to control pain and sleeplessness)

   e. The type of food and fluids that the patient may have (typically, the patient has ice chips and sips of water to determine if nausea or vomiting are likely to occur)

   f. The recording of intake and output

   g. Care of the wound

   h. The frequency and positions in which the patient is to be turned

   i. The time dangling and ambulation should be started

   j. Laboratory examinations to be done immediately or on the day following surgery

CHAPTER 28

Wound Care

The number in parentheses following each rationale indicates on which page in *Fundamental Skills and Concepts in Patient Care,* Seventh Edition, you can find the correct answer.

ANSWERS TO MATCHING QUESTIONS

Items 1 Through 6

(Refer to Table 28-1, page 592)

1. (g)
2. (c)
3. (f)
4. (a)
5. (e)
6. (b)

Items 7 Through 9

(Refer to page 603)

7. (d)
8. (c)
9. (a)

ANSWERS TO MULTIPLE CHOICE QUESTIONS

Items 1 Through 15

1. (d)   The sequence of activities associated with the inflammatory process are swelling, pain, decreased functioning, redness, and warmth.   (592)
2. (a)   The components of a scab are cells called fibroblasts and a substance called collagen. These two act as building blocks and "glue" to temporarily repair the area that was damaged.   (592)
3. (c)   Wound healing involves the body's efforts to restore the structure and function of cells in the in-

jured area. This is done either by recovery of injured cells, called *resolution;* by replacement of damaged cells with identical new cells, called *regeneration;* or by the production of a nonfunctioning substitute for the destroyed cells, called *scar formation.*   (592)

4. (c)   *Granulation tissue* is pinkish-red tissue containing new projections of capillaries.   (592)
5. (d)   Careful handwashing before caring for the wound probably is the *single most* effective method of preventing infections. (Review Asepsis)
6. (d)   The primary cause of a pressure sore is unrelieved compression of capillaries bringing blood to the skin and its underlying tissue. The mechanism for destruction is as follows: The body weight compresses the tissue and blood vessels against the hard surface of a bed, chair, bedpan, and so on. As a result, the cells supplied through the vascular network lack oxygen and a means for carrying away waste products of metabolism. Cells eventually die if these conditions are prolonged and unrelieved.   (602)
7. (d)   The earliest sign of excessive pressure is a red appearance to the skin over a bony area of the body. The color is due to cellular damage in the area.   (603)
8. (c)   Refer to Focus on Older Adults, page 606 and Display 28-2, page 604.
9. (a)   One of the common purposes of dressing a wound is to absorb drainage.   (594)
10. (c)   If changing a dressing is likely to be a painful experience for the patient, the nurse should give a prescribed medication about 15 to 30 minutes before a dressing change to reduce discomfort. (Skill 28-1 page 608)
11. (b)   Staples have an advantage in that they are less likely to compress tissue if a wound swells. This is prevented because staples do not encircle the wound; they merely form a bridge that holds the two sides together.   (596)

12. (b)   The wound heals toward the center; pulling the wound edge could reinjure healing tissue. (Skill 28-1) page 608

13. (a)   A solution for an eye irritation should be approximately body temperature.   (578)

14. (d)   Older adults are often insensitive to hot and cold applications. Consequently, they are at great risk for sustaining thermal injuries.   (588)

15. (c)   The purpose of the spiral-reverse turn method of bandaging is to bandage a cone-shaped body part, such as the thigh or leg.   (597)

ANSWERS TO TRUE OR FALSE QUESTIONS

Items 1 Through 12

1. *False.* Second intention is a type of wound healing in which widely separated edges of a wound must heal inward toward the center. First intention healing is when the wound edges are directly next to one another.   (593)

2. *False.* Third intention is a type of wound healing in which temporarily separated wound edges are eventually brought together at a later time.   (593)

3. *True.*

4. *False.* Shearing force is the damaging effect that occurs when compressed layers of tissue move upon each other.   (604)

5. *True.*

6. *False.* During the prevention and treatment of a closed pressure sore, the focus is on keeping the area dry. When the skin is broken, the nurse must maintain a moist environment. Moisture promotes the movement of epidermal cells to the surface of the wound, causing it to seal over and heal. (Text Chapter 28)

7. *False.* Prevention of additional injury and the promotion of healing are two principal goals of wound care.   (592)

8. *False.* Perhaps the best feature of transparent dressings is that they allow assessment without removing the dressing.   (595)

9. *True.*

10. *False.* Any wound irrigation that is performed in a body area that contains intact tissue will not necessarily need to follow principles of sterile technique. However, when an irrigation is required for an incision or other open wound, surgical asepsis should be followed. (Skill 28-2)

11. *False.* The drainage basin used to collect the solution from an irrigation need not be sterile, since it will receive solution contaminated with organisms and debris from the irrigated area.   (599)

12. *False.* If the item is a bean, pea, or similar dehydrated substance, irrigation is contraindicated. The solution can cause it to swell and become fixed even more tightly than before. Solid objects are likely to require removal with an instrument. An exception would be in the case of a live insect. The insect can be suffocated by instilling and briefly retaining water or oil within the auditory canal. The dead insect will usually pass out as the fluid drains from the ear.   (600)

ANSWERS TO SHORT ANSWER QUESTIONS

Items 1 Through 6

1. The sequence of events that are associated with the inflammatory process are (refer to pages 592–593):
   a. The injured cells release chemical substances that set the inflammation in motion.
   b. White blood cells, called neutrophils and monocytes, are drawn to the injured area and begin to engulf dead cells and debris.
   c. Once the area has been cleaned, cells called fibroblasts and a substance called collagen fill the injured area.
   d. The body begins to send new projections of capillaries into the area to supply replacement cells with oxygen and nutrients.

2. Common purposes of dressing a wound are (refer to page 594):
   a. To help keep a wound clean and restrict entry of organisms
   b. To absorb drainage
   c. To control edema and bleeding when applied with pressure
   d. To protect the healing area from further injury
   e. To help hold antiseptic medication next to the wound
   f. Maintain a moist environment

3. Equipment and supplies suggested for a dressing change are (refer to Skill 28-1, page 608):
   a. A sterile cloth or paper on which to set up a sterile field
   b. Forceps or clean gloves to handle soiled dressing
   c. Sterile forceps and a pair of sterile gloves with which to apply sterile dressing materials
   d. A sterile cup for antiseptic solution
   e. A special solvent if spray-on adhesive has been used
   f. Sterile normal saline in case the dressing sticks to the wound

g. A waterproof bag to receive the soiled dressing
h. Dressings of various sizes
i. Tape for securing the dressing

4. Nursing measures when caring for a wound with a drain are (refer to pages 595 and 596):
   a. Assess the characteristics and amount of the drainage.
   b. Cleanse the area around the drain.
   c. Clean the skin around the drain using circular motions.
   d. Shorten the drain by using a gentle twisting motion. Cut the excess length and replace the safety pin or clamp near the end of the drain.
   e. Remove the drain using the same twisting motion as in shortening.

5. Recommended techniques for securing a dressing are (refer to pages 594–597):
   a. Plan to use adhesive or paper tape for most dressings.
   b. Consider shaving the area if necessary.
   c. Remove adhesive remnants before applying new tape.
   d. Fold under each end of an adhesive strip to create a tab.
   e. Apply a protective coating to the skin.

f. Moisten adhesive with a little alcohol if it does not stick to the skin easily.
g. Try using liquid adhesive for small areas.
h. Do not cover the entire surface of the dressing with tape.
i. Observe the patient for sensitivity to tape.
j. Use Montgomery straps for large areas that may need changing often.
k. Exert pressure on the wound from the edges toward the center of the wound when securing a dressing.
l. Secure the dressing snugly so that it does not slip.
m. Use protection if there is drainage.
n. Consider using a binder or bandage when adhesive tape is impractical.

6. Purposes of bandages and binders are (refer to page 597):
   a. They can be used to hold dressings in place.
   b. They prevent tension on sutures when properly applied.
   c. They permit motion in order to promote healing.
   d. They can be used to provide support for a body part.
   e. They provide comfort and a sense of security for the patient.

Gastrointestinal Intubation

The number in parentheses following each rationale indicates on which page in *Fundamental Skills and Concepts in Patient Care,* Seventh Edition, you can find the correct answer.

ANSWERS TO MATCHING QUESTIONS

Items 1 Through 6

(Refer to Table 29-1, page 619)

1.	(c)	4.	(d)
2.	(e)	5.	(f)
3.	(b)	6.	(a)

Items 7 Through 10

(Refer to Table 29-3, page 627)

7.	(b)	9.	(a)
8.	(d)	10.	(c)

Items 11 Through 20

(Refer to Table 29-5, page 630)

11.	(d)	16.	(g)
12.	(i)	17.	(j)
13.	(a)	18.	(e)
14.	(f)	19.	(b)
15.	(h)	20.	(c)

ANSWERS TO MULTIPLE CHOICE QUESTIONS

Items 1 Through 15

1. (d)   One of the common causes of diarrhea associated with tube feedings is a formula that is highly concentrated. (See Table 29-5, page 630)

2. (a)   Constipation is often a problem associated with tube feedings that lack fiber. (See Table 29-5, page 630)

3. (b)   To maintain tube patency, it is best to flush feeding tubes with 30 to 60 ml of water immediately before and after administering a feeding or medication; every four hours if the patient has continuous feedings; and after refeeding the gastric residual. (Skill 29–4, pages 644)

4. (d)   Other than being inserted into the nose, a tube can be inserted through the skin and tissue of the abdomen and secured with gastrointestinal sutures. This method, called a transabdominal tube, is used in lieu of nasogastric or nasointestinal tubes when patients require an alternative to oral feeding for longer than a month.   (629)

5. (c)   The process of removing a poisonous substance through gastric intubation is called lavage.   (618)

6. (b)   A common cause of feeding-tube obstruction is administering formula at rates less than 50 ml/hr.   (629)

7. (a)   One of the advantages of the nasogastric tube is that it has a low incidence of obstruction. (See Table 29-3, page 627)

8. (d)   An advantage of the gastrostomy over other feeding tubes is that it can remain in place for up to 4 weeks. (See Table 29-3, page 627)

9. (c)   The Ewald orogastric tube has a diameter of 36 to 40 French, the largest of the gastrointestinal tubes. (See Table 29-1, page 619)

10. (a)   A bolus feeding is the instillation of a large volume of liquid nourishment into the stomach in a fairly short amount of time.   (627)

11. (c)   Most formulas used for tube feedings provide 0.5 to 2.0 kcal/ml of formula.   (627)

12. (d)   Bolus feedings are the least desirable because they distend the stomach rapidly, causing gastric discomfort and the risk for reflux and aspiration to occur.   (627)

13. (b)   Gastric residual is the volume of liquid within the stomach after allowing a compensatory time for stomach emptying.   (628)

14. (a)   Despite the fact that tube feedings are approximately 80% water, patients generally require more. Adults require 30 ml/kg of weight or 1 ml/kcal on a daily basis.   (629)

15. (a)   Instilling a tube feeding too rapidly can result in nausea and vomiting. (See Table 29-5, page 630)

ANSWERS TO TRUE OR FALSE QUESTIONS

Items 1 Through 10

1. *True.*
2. *True.*
3. *False.* Transabdominal tubes are used in lieu of nasogastric or nasointestinal tubes when the patient requires an alternative to oral feeding for longer than a month.   (620)
4. *True.*
5. *False.* Place the tip of the nasogastric tube at the end of the nose, then to the earlobe, and finally to the xiphoid process of the sternum. This is referred to as the NEX (nose-earlobe-xiphoid) measurement. It approximates the length of tubing required to reach the stomach.   (621)
6. *True.*
7. *False.* Never reinsert the stylet while the tube is in the patient. The stylet can puncture the flexible tube and injure the body structures where it protrudes.   (624)
8. *True.*

9. *False.* Intestinal decompression refers to the removal of gas and fluids from the small bowel.   (620)

10. *False.* If the gastrostomy becomes accidentally extubated, the nurse may insert a Foley catheter 5 to 10 cm into the opening and inflate the balloon to maintain patency until re-intubation can be accomplished.   (626)

ANSWERS TO SHORT ANSWER QUESTIONS

Items 1 Through 4

1. Methods for determining if a nasogastric tube is in the stomach are (refer to page 622):
   a. Aspirating fluid—fluid appears clear, brownish-yellow, or green
   b. Auscultating the abdomen—instill 10 ml or more of air; listen with a stethoscope over the abdomen. You will hear a swooshing sound as air enters the stomach.
   c. Testing the *p*H of aspirated fluid—most definitive method. Stomach fluid is acid with a *p*H of 1 to 3.

2. Steps to follow for administering an intermittent feeding are (refer to Skill 29-4, page 642):
   a. Fill container with room temperature formula.
   b. Purge air from the tubing by gradually opening the clamp on the tube.
   c. Connect tubing to the nasogastric or nasoenteral tube.
   d. Open the clamp and regulate the drip according to the physician's order.
   e. Check at 10-minute intervals.
   f. Flush tubing with water after formula has infused.
   g. Pinch the nasal tube just as the last of the volume of water is given.
   h. Clamp or plug the nasal tube.
   i. Record the volume of formula and water instilled.
   j. Keep the head of the bed elevated for at least 30 to 60 minutes after a feeding.
   k. Record the volume of formula and water administered on the intake and output record.
   l. Provide oral hygiene at least twice daily.

3. Four schedules for administering tube feedings are (refer to pages 627–628):
   a. A bolus feeding is the instillation of a large volume of liquid nourishment in a fairly short amount of time. Approximately 250 to 400 ml of formula are given over a few minutes. They are repeated four to six times a day.
   b. An intermittent feeding is the instillation of liquid nourishment into the stomach in the time most people would spend eating a meal. Usually the volume is 250 to 400 ml. They are usually given by gravity drip over 30 to 60 minutes. Feedings are repeated four to six times a day.
   c. A cyclic feeding is one that is given continuously for 8 to 12 hours followed by a 1- to 12-hour pause. This routine is often used to wean patients while providing adequate nutrition. The feeding is given during the late evening hours and during sleep.
   d. A continuous feeding is the instillation of a small volume of liquid nourishment without any interruption. Approximately 1.5 ml/minute is administered. An electric feeding pump is used to regulate the infusion. This type of feeding may be administered directly into the small intestine.

4. Purposes for gastrointestinal intubation are (refer to page 618):
   a. Provide nourishment
   b. Administer oral medications that cannot be swallowed
   c. Obtain samples of secretions for diagnostic testing
   d. Remove poisonous substances
   e. Remove gas and secretions from the stomach or bowel
   f. Control gastric bleeding

CHAPTER 30

Urinary Elimination

The number in parentheses following each rationale indicates on which page in *Fundamental Skills and Concepts in Patient Care,* Seventh Edition, you can find the correct answer.

ANSWERS TO MATCHING QUESTIONS

Items 1 Through 5

(Refer to Table 30-2, page 656)

1. (e)
2. (d)
3. (f)
4. (a)
5. (c)

Items 6 Through 10

(Refer to Table 30-2, page 656)

6. (b)
7. (f)
8. (a)
9. (e)
10. (c)

ANSWERS TO MULTIPLE CHOICE QUESTIONS

Items 1 Through 12

1. (c) The kidneys perform the major responsibility for maintaining the balance of water and other chemicals in blood and cells. The blood delivers these substances to microscopic structures called nephrons in the kidneys. The nephrons selectively remove excess water and substances for which the body has no need, forming urine. (652)

2. (b) As the volume of urine increases, the bladder expands and pressure increases within it. When the pressure becomes sufficient to stimulate stretch receptors located in the bladder wall, the desire to empty the bladder becomes noticeable. Usually, this occurs in adults when about 150 to 300 ml of urine collects in the bladder. (652)

3. (a) *Anuria* refers to the absence of urine. (654)

4. (d) *Urinary suppression* indicates that the kidneys are not forming urine. *Oliguria* is the production of a small volume of urine, usually less than 400 ml of urine in 24 hours when oral intake has been adequate and no other excessive amount of fluid has been lost. *Anuria* refers to the absence of urine. Because the kidneys are not producing urine, the bladder remains empty. (654)

5. (b) Residual urine is urine retained in the bladder after a patient voids. *Urinary retention* means that urine is being produced but is not being emptied from the bladder. *Urinary incontinence* is the inability to control the release of urine from the bladder. (654)

6. (b) Stress incontinence is a condition in which small amounts of urine are released from the bladder only at times when there is increased abdominal pressure, such as when coughing or sneezing. (Refer to Table 30-2, page 656)

7. (a) Approximately 500 ml to 2500 ml of urine in each 24-hour period is excreted by the healthy adult. The average is about 1200 ml. (Table 30-1, 653)

8. (c) The term for pus in the urine is *pyuria.* (654)

9. (c) Strengthening pelvic floor muscles is one method for controlling some types of incontinence. It is especially helpful for stress incontinence and may extend the time needed for control in urge incontinence. The pelvic floor muscle exercises, also called Kegel exercises, increase the tone of the pubococcygeus muscles. (657)

10. (b)   The procedure of catheterization is used as infrequently as possible due to the hazards involved. Only when the benefits outweigh the risks should the nurse propose to insert a catheter. The nurse should also advocate for its early removal.   (655)

11. (c)   A *straight catheter* is a hollow tube that is intended to be inserted and withdrawn following its use for some temporary measure. An *indwelling catheter* is one that is placed into the bladder and secured there for a period of time. It is sometimes called a retention catheter. The most commonly used indwelling catheter is called a *Foley catheter*.   (658)

12. (a)   When an external catheter is used, there are certain potential problems that may occur. First, and perhaps the most hazardous, is that the appliance may be applied too tightly and restrict blood flow to the skin and tissues of the penis. Second, moisture accumulates beneath the appliance and this can lead to breakdown of the skin covering the penis. Third, the catheter may not fit well or for some other reason lead to leaking of urine.   (658)

ANSWERS TO TRUE OR FALSE QUESTIONS

Items 1 Through 12

1. *False.* The urethra is the final passageway for urine as it is released from the bladder. The urine is transported from the kidneys through the ureters to the urinary bladder.   (652)
2. *True.*
3. *False. Oliguria* refers to the production of only small amounts of urine. *Anuria* refers to the absence of urine.   (654)
4. *False. Polyuria* means an excessive production and excretion of urine. The term for blood in the urine is *hematuria.*   (654)
5. *False.* A catheter that drains well does not need irrigating, except on rare occasions when irrigation is used to instill medications.   (660)
6. *False.* Seeing to it that the patient with an indwelling catheter has a generous fluid intake increases urine production and dilutes particles that may form in the urine.   (663)
7. *True.*
8. *False.* Catheterizations that are performed in health agencies follow principles of surgical asepsis. Self-catheterization is done following principles of medical asepsis.   (659)
9. *True.*

10. *False.* A clean-catch midstream specimen is a voided specimen collected under conditions of thorough cleanliness and after a small amount of urine is voided into the toilet.   (653)
11. *True.*
12. *False.* Incontinent patients should be instructed that limiting fluid intake is a dangerous method to control urination.   (663)

ANSWERS TO SHORT ANSWER QUESTIONS

Items 1 Through 4

1. Actions that are helpful when the male patient uses the urinal are (refer to page 655):
   a. Make sure the urinal is empty before handing it to the patient.
   b. Warm the metal urinal with water.
   c. Instruct the patient to spread his legs if he cannot place the urinal himself.
   d. While holding the handle of the urinal, direct it at an angle between the patient's legs so that the bottom rests on the bed.
   e. Lift the penis and place it well within the inside of the urinal.
2. Bladder retraining plans could be (refer to pages 656–657):
   a. Assess for any patterns of dryness versus incontinence.
   b. Set realistic goals.
   c. Plan a specific schedule and be sure all personnel carry it out.
   d. Discourage strict limitation of liquid intake.
   e. Be sure all personnel, family, and any others know the planned schedule.
   f. Teach the patient to note any sensation that precedes voiding.
   g. Encourage a relaxed atmosphere and as near normal circumstances.
   h. Suggest that the patient bend forward in a slow, rhythmic manner.
   i. Experiment with the success of measures to stimulate urination, such as listening to running water or placing the hands in water.

3. Factors that influence the amount, contents, and characteristics of urine or its elimination are (refer to pages 652–653):
   a. The amount of urine normally produced varies with the fluid intake. The greater the intake, the larger the output and vice versa.
   b. Contents and character are related to the individuals diet and the chemical composition of body fluids.
   c. Frequency depends on the amount of urine produced.
   d. The intervals of voiding are generally due to habit.
   e. Increased abdominal pressure can increase the urge to void.
   f. Stress, embarrassment, even sometimes the need for a urine specimen can cause the patient difficulty in relaxing enough to void.
   g. Women void most easily in a semisitting or sitting position and men find it easiest to void in the standing position.

4. The following nursing measures should be kept in mind when the patient needs assistance with urination (refer to pages 654–657):
   a. Provide privacy. Voiding may not occur if the patient is tense or worried about being observed or interrupted.
   b. Help females to assume a sitting position. Sitting is the natural position women assume for elimination.
   c. Assist males to stand in front of a toilet or stand at the bedside when using a urinal. Standing is the natural position men assume when urinating.
   d. Maintain an adequate intake of oral fluids. The urge to urinate is dependent on the pressure exerted against stretch receptors as the bladder fills.

CHAPTER 31

Bowel Elimination

The number in parentheses following each rationale indicates on which page in *Fundamental Skills and Concepts in Patient Care,* Seventh Edition, you can find the correct answer.

ANSWERS TO MATCHING QUESTIONS

Items 1 Through 8

(Refer to pages 685–686.)

1. (b)
2. (c)
3. (a)
4. (b)
5. (a)
6. (c)
7. (c)
8. (a)

ANSWERS TO MULTIPLE CHOICE QUESTIONS

Items 1 Through 20

1. (b) The volume of the stool is affected by the amount of food that is consumed. A diet high in fiber and roughage produces a larger stool and promotes quicker passage through the intestinal tract. A diet low in roughage produces a smaller stool and tends to increase the time it remains within the bowel. (685)

2. (c) Constipation is a condition in which the stool becomes dry and hard and requires straining in order to eliminate it. The frequency of stool passage is not always a factor. Some persons may be constipated and yet have a daily bowel movement. (685)

3. (b) A patient with a fecal impaction may expel liquid stool around the impacted mass. This symptom in combination with a lack of normal defecation is almost a sure indication of an impaction. (686)

4. (c) Several measures may relieve a fecal impaction. The stool may be passed if sufficient moisture and lubrication are instilled into the rectum in the area of the stool. An oil retention enema is often prescribed to first provide lubrication to the mass and the mucous membrane that lines the rectum. (686)

5. (d) Digital removal of stool may become necessary if the administration of enemas fails to produce results for the patient with a fecal impaction. Digital removal involves inserting a gloved and well-lubricated finger into the rectum in order to break up and remove the fecal mass. (686)

6. (b) An excessive amount of gas within the intestinal tract is known as *flatulence.* Expelled intestinal gas is called *flatus.* When gas is not expelled and instead accumulates, the condition is called *intestinal distention* or *tympanites.* (687)

7. (c) The largest percentage of gas accumulated in the bowel comes from swallowed air and the air that is present in food. Other minor sources include gas that diffuses from the bloodstream and bacterial fermentation. (687)

8. (c) Insert a rectal tube to help gas escape. Gas will usually follow the path of least resistance. The inserted tube provides a channel through which the gas can travel. An intestinal tube inserted through the nose may be used as a last resort. (687)

9. (d) Diarrhea is the passage of watery, unformed stools accompanied by abdominal cramping. Although frequent bowel movements do not necessarily mean that diarrhea is present, persons with diarrhea usually have stools frequently. (687)

10. (c)   To help the patient who has diarrhea, the nurse should temporarily limit the consumption of food. Provide clear liquids until the number of stools and the consistency improve and then follow with bananas, applesauce, and light foods. Avoid fried foods, highly seasoned foods, or foods high in roughage.   (687)

11. (b)   Anal control is dependent ultimately on proper functioning of the anal sphincters. For some patients, functioning of impaired sphincters can be improved. One way is to consult with the physician about using a suppository or an enema every 2 to 3 days. If a pattern can be established by stimulating peristalsis and emptying the lower bowel with these aids, fecal incontinence may become controllable.   (687)

12. (a)   Defecation usually occurs within 5 to 15 minutes after administration of a large-volume enema.   (688)

13. (c)   Tap water or normal saline are preferred for their nonirritating effect on patients. However, tap water can be absorbed through the bowel. Tap water enemas that are repeated one after another can result in fluid imbalances.   (688)

14. (d)   A hypertonic solution is one in which there is a higher amount of dissolved substances than that found in the blood. Hypertonic enema solutions act by increasing fluid volume in the intestine and by acting as a local irritant.   (688)

15. (c)   The recommended position for the patient receiving a hypertonic enema is the knee-chest position. This position allows for good distribution of solution to the lower large intestine.   (688)

16. (a)   The primary purpose of an oil retention enema is to lubricate and soften the stool so that it can be expelled more easily.   (689)

17. (d)   Prevention of skin breakdown is one of the biggest challenges in ostomy care. Enzymes in stool can quickly cause excoriation.   (689)

18. (d)   When the patient is elderly, assess intestinal elimination patterns accurately. Many elderly persons become very bowel conscious and report a problem with constipation erroneously because they lack accurate information concerning elimination.   (693)

19. (b)   Although laxatives and enemas sometimes play a proper role in intestinal elimination, they are also very often abused. Teaching their proper use and the dangers of abuse is a nursing responsibility.   (686)

20. (a)   The gastrocolic reflex generally precedes defecation.   (684)

ANSWERS TO TRUE OR FALSE QUESTIONS

Items 1 Through 12

1. *False.* The *external* anal sphincter is under voluntary control.   (Refer to Table 31-1, page 684)
2. *True.*
3. *False.* Constipation is a condition in which the stool becomes hard and dry and requires straining to eliminate it. The frequency of stool passage is not always a factor.   (685)
4. *True.*
5. *True.*
6. *True.*
7. *False.* Consuming gas-forming foods increases the volume of gas in the intestinal tract.   (687)
8. *False.* Diarrhea is the passage of watery, unformed stools accompanied by abdominal cramping. Although frequent bowel movements do not necessarily mean that diarrhea is present, persons with diarrhea usually have stools frequently.   (687)
9. *False.* A hypertonic enema solution will cause fluid to be drawn from body tissues into the bowel, eventually increasing the fluid volume in the intestine to more than the original amount that was instilled.   (688)
10. *False.* An ileostomy is an opening into the ileum, a portion of the small intestine.   (689–690)
11. *True.*
12. *True.*

ANSWERS TO SHORT ANSWER QUESTIONS

Items 1 Through 5

1. The conditions that predispose a person to form greater amounts of gas or interfere with its absorption include   (refer to page 687):
   a. Swallowing larger than usual amounts of air while eating and drinking.
   b. As a by-product of bacterial fermentation.
   c. Consuming gas-forming foods increases the volume of gas in the intestinal tract.
   d. Inactivity tends to impair the movement of gas through the intestinal tract.
   e. Some patients experience intestinal distention after surgery in which the bowel is handled.
   f. Drugs such as morphine tend to decrease peristalsis and thus cause distention as well as constipation.
   g. The presence of a mass that obstructs the passage of stool may also interfere with the ability of the intestine to eliminate gas.

2. The chief characteristics of constipation include   (refer to page 695):
   a. Abdominal distention or bloating
   b. Change in the amount of gas passed rectally
   c. Less frequent bowel movements
   d. Oozing liquid stool
   e. Rectal fullness or pressure
   f. Rectal pain with bowel movement
   g. Small amount of stool
   h. Unable to pass stool
3. Causes of diarrhea are (refer to page 687):
   a. The response of the body to try and rid itself of some allergic substance or the natural defense for eliminating an irritating substance such as tainted food or intestinal pathogens
   b. The response to stress
   c. Certain dietary indiscretions
   d. Intentional or accidental abuse of laxatives
   e. Many intestinal and digestive diseases
4. Nursing measures suggested to help relieve diarrhea are (refer to page (687):
   a. Remember that diarrhea is often an embarrassing situation.
   b. Reduce the cause if possible.
   c. Temporarily limit food and then start by providing clear liquids. Give nonirritating foods and avoid fried foods and foods high in roughage.
   d. Investigate the relationship between side effects of medications and the occurrence of diarrhea.
   e. Remember that individuals with diarrhea find it very difficult to delay the urge to defecate.
   f. Use hygienic measures to clean the perineum following each stool.
   g. Count the number of stools the patient is having.
   h. Consult with the physician concerning the possible use of medications to control the diarrhea.
5. Causes of fecal incontinence are (refer to page 687):
   a. It is usually the result of disease or injury.
   b. A fecal impaction may be present.
   c. It may be a temporary loss of control.
   d. Waiting for the bedpan or the use of a toilet causes some individuals to have loss of control.
   e. Taking an extremely harsh or large dosage of a laxative may result in rapid peristalsis.

CHAPTER 32

Oral Medications

The number in parentheses following each rationale indicates on which page in *Fundamental Skills and Concepts in Patient Care,* Seventh Edition, you can find the correct answer.

ANSWERS TO MATCHING QUESTIONS

Items 1 Through 6

(Refer to page 711)

1. (d)
2. (c)
3. (f)
4. (h)
5. (g)
6. (b)

Items 7 Through 10

(Refer to Table 32-1, page 710)

7. (c)
8. (d)
9. (b)
10. (a)

ANSWERS TO MULTIPLE CHOICE QUESTIONS

Items 1 Through 12

1. (b) The trade, or proprietary, name is the name used by the manufacturer for the drug it sells. The drug's generic, or nonproprietary, name is a name that is usually descriptive of the drug's chemical structure and is not protected by a company's trademark. (710)

2. (c) Medication errors are serious! A medication order should *never* be implemented if the nurse has a question about it until after consulting the physician or another authorized person. (710)

3. (c) Most health care agencies check narcotic supplies at the change of shifts. A nurse completing one shift checks the narcotic count with a nurse beginning the next shift. (713)

4. (b) For many years, nurses have followed five criteria for assuring that medications are prepared and administered correctly. These criteria have been described as the FIVE RIGHTS for administering medication. The FIVE RIGHTS are:
   1. The Right Drug
   2. The Right Dose
   3. The Right Route
   4. The Right Time
   5. The Right Patient   (713)

5. (b) The nurse should check the label of the drug container *three* times to ensure safety and accuracy: (1) when reaching for the medication; (2) immediately prior to pouring the medication; and (3) when returning the container to its storage place.   (714)

6. (d) When administering medications, the nurse should remain with the patient while he takes the medication. Do not leave medications at the bedside for the patient to take at a later time. The patient may forget to take the medication or some else may take it.   (714)

7. (a) Do not give a medication without further checking if the patient indicates that the drug appears different from what he has been receiving. A mistake may have been made when supplying the medication or when preparing the medication. Withholding it while checking further may avoid an error.   (713)

8. (d) If a medication error occurs, the patient's condition is checked and the error is reported to the physician and the supervising nurse immediately.   (716)

9. (c)   Certain tablets are covered with a substance that does not dissolve until the medication reaches the small intestine. These tablets are enteric coated. If the coating is destroyed, the medication is released in the stomach, where it is irritating to the gastric mucosa. Enteric-coated tablets should never be crushed or chewed.   (710)

10. (c)   One of the main reasons the nurse should stay with the patient until the oral medication is swallowed is that the nurse is responsible for documenting that the drug was taken by the patient. It is possible that a patient could discard a drug, misplace it, or accumulate many in order to harm himself.   (715).

11. (b)   If the nasogastric tube is used for suctioning rather than nourishment, the tube must be clamped for at least a half hour after instilling medication. If that is not done, the drugs are removed from the stomach before they can be absorbed.   (722)

12. (c)   Monitor the elderly person's medication carefully while taking into account the effects of aging. As a result of aging, the risk of adverse side effects and toxicity to drugs increases. Decreased gastrointestinal motility and decreased ability to absorb drugs tend to reduce the drug action because the drugs are not being taken into the bloodstream as well.   (718)

ANSWERS TO TRUE OR FALSE QUESTIONS

Items 1 Through 12

1. *True.*
2. *False.* Clerical activities may be delegated, but the nurse is the one responsible within a health agency for checking, transcribing, and carrying out the medication order.   (pages 710–711)
3. *False.* The trade or proprietary name is the name used by the manufacturer for the drug it sells. The drug's generic or nonproprietary name is a name that is usually descriptive of the drug's chemical structure and is not protected by a company's trademark.   (710)
4. *True.*
5. *False.* A drug that is ordered to be given four times a day may be scheduled in a variety of patterns. For example, it may be given at: 8 A.M., 12 noon, 4 P.M., and 8 P.M.; or 10 A.M., 2 P.M., 6 P.M., and 10 P.M.; or 6 A.M., 12 noon, 6 P.M., and 12 midnight.   (711)
6. *False.* Federal law requires that a record be kept for each narcotic that is administered.   (713)
7. *True.*

8. *False.* There is a sixth RIGHT some nurses have added to the list. It is the patient's right to refuse medication. The right of a rational adult patient to consent to or refuse therapy is a legal right.   (713)
9. *False.* Health care agencies have a special form for reporting medication errors, called an *incident sheet* or *accident report.* In this report, a full explanation of the situation is provided. The report serves as a method for preventing future errors by examining the practices that contributed to the error. The incident sheet is *not* a part of the patient's permanent record, nor should any reference be made in the chart that an incident sheet has been completed.   (716)
10. *False.* A notation should be made stating why the medication was not given as scheduled. This is not considered a medication error in most instances.   (716)
11. *False.* Medications should not be added to the formula being administered for continuous tube feedings.   (715)
12. *False.* Enteric-coated tablets or those designed for sustained release should never be crushed and administered. This interferes with their absorption and the desired therapeutic effects.   (715)

ANSWERS TO SHORT ANSWER QUESTIONS

Items 1 Through 5

1. The seven parts of a complete medication order are (refer to page 710):
   a. The name of the patient
   b. The date and time the order is written
   c. The name of the medication
   d. The dosage to be administered
   e. The route for administering medication
   f. The frequency of administering the medication
   g. The signature of the person who has written the order
2. The five items of information the nurse should know about the patient before administering medications are (text, Chapter 32).
   a. Nonprescription medications the patient uses and the reason, frequency, and length of time he has been using them
   b. Prescription medications that the patient has been using and the reason, frequency, and length of time he has been using them
   c. The patient's pattern for following the directions for medication use
   d. Any allergies the patient has to medications
   e. The patient's habits of daily living that may influence drug therapy, such as alcohol and drug consumption

3. The FIVE RIGHTS pertaining to administering medications are (refer to page 713):
   a. The Right Drug
   b. The Right Dose
   c. The Right Route
   d. The Right Time
   e. The Right Patient
4. The five steps that the nurse should carry out prior to preparing drugs that will be administered are (throughout the text):
   a. Check the patient's medication record with the original medication orders prior to preparing the drugs.
   b. Question any part of a drug order that appears inappropriate before proceeding.
   c. Be alert to any unusual changes, such as new additions or deletions, of entries on the medication record. Errors can occur when forms are recopied or when transcribing a new medication order.
   d. Question any unusual abbreviations that may have been used when transcribing a medication order. Errors have occurred when the person writing the order or transcribing is has used unacceptable abbreviations. This practice can cause misinterpretation when administering the medication.
   e. Organize the nursing care so that medications are given as near to the scheduled routine as possible. It is common policy to give the drug no earlier or later than 30 minutes from the time specified. A medication given outside this range of time is considered a drug error.

5. Guidelines the nurse should follow when preparing medications for administration are (refer to page 714):
   a. Prepare medications while using a good light, and work alone without interruptions or distractions. Also, allow sufficient time so that all the drugs may be prepared without having to leave and return to complete the task.
   b. Check the label of the drug container *three* times to ensure safety and accuracy: (1) when reaching for the medication; (2) immediately prior to pouring the medication; and (3) when returning the container to its storage place.
   c. Do not use medications from containers on which the label is difficult to read or has come off.
   d. Do not return medications to a container or transfer medications from one container to another.
   e. Check expiration dates on medications, especially those that are in solution. Do not use a medication that has a sediment at the bottom of the container unless the medication is to be shaken well before using. Do not use one that appears cloudy or has changed color.
   f. Prepare medications in the order in which they will be delivered to patients.
   g. Transport drugs from the area of preparation to the patient carefully and safely. Use the method of transporting provided by the agency. Identify the drugs in some manner to avoid confusing which drugs are for which patients.
   h. Protect needles for injecting drugs according to the method of the agency's choice to prevent contamination.
   i. Use an individual medicine dropper for each liquid medication dispensed in this manner.

CHAPTER 33

Topical and Inhalant Medications

The number in parentheses following each rationale indicates on which page in *Fundamental Skills and Concepts in Patient Care,* Seventh Edition, you can find the correct answer.

ANSWERS TO MATCHING QUESTIONS

Items 1 Through 5

(Refer to Table 33-1, page 726)

1. (e)
2. (c)
3. (a)
4. (b)
5. (d)

ANSWERS TO MULTIPLE CHOICE QUESTIONS

Items 1 Through 10

1. (a) To ensure good absorption when applying an inunction, the nurse should first cleanse the area with soap or detergent and water before applying the oil, lotion, cream, or ointment. This frees the skin of debris and body oil, both of which retard absorption. (726)
2. (c) Do not touch the ointment. The medication can be absorbed through any skin surface. (727)
3. (b) When administering ear drops to an adult, gently pull the ear upward and backward. (727)
4. (d) When administering ear drops to a child, gently pull the ear downward and backward. (727)
5. (b) Some medications are intended to become absorbed through the blood vessels within the mouth rather than be delivered to the gastrointestinal tract. A sublingual administration involves placing a drug under the tongue. A buccal adminis-tration involves placing a drug against the mucous membranes of the cheek. (728)
6. (c) The position of choice when inserting a vaginal medication is the dorsal recumbent position with the knees flexed and slightly spread upon the bed. (728)
7. (a) The mucous membrane of the eye is called the conjunctiva. (727)
8. (c) If medication is to be instilled in both ears, it is appropriate to wait 15 minutes before instilling the medication in the other ear. (728)
9. (d) Chewing and swallowing the pill, smoking, eating, and drinking are all contraindicated when a buccal medication has been given. (728)
10. (b) When inserting medications vaginally with an applicator, one should follow the package directions, which usually recommend inserting the applicator about 2 to 4 inches into the vagina. (728)

ANSWERS TO TRUE OR FALSE QUESTIONS

Items 1 Through 9

1. *False.* Topically applied drugs may have a local or systemic effect. (725)
2. *False.* Clip, but do not shave, body hair that will be covered by the patch. Shaving creates microabrasions that could increase the rate of drug absorption. Clipping reduces the discomfort during patch removal. (725)
3. *True.*
4. *True.*
5. *False.* It is important to monitor the heart rate and blood pressure of older adults who use inhalers containing bronchodilating drugs. These types of medications often cause tachycardia and hypotension. (Refer to Focus on Older Adults, page 731)
6. *True.*

336

7. *True.*
8. *True.*
9. *False.* Cutaneous applications are those in which topical drugs are applied to the skin. An *inunction* is a medication that is incorporated into a transporting agent. All inunctions are cutaneous applications but not all cutaneous applications are inunctions. (725)

ANSWERS TO SHORT ANSWER QUESTIONS

Items 1 Through 4

1. The seven guidelines for giving an inunction are (refer to page 726):
   a. Cleanse the skin and hands with soap or detergent and water before applying the oil, lotion, cream, or ointment.
   b. Shake the contents of mixtures that may have become separated.
   c. Apply most inunctions with the fingers and hands or use a cotton ball or gauze square.
   d. Wear gloves if there is a contagious skin condition or there are breaks in the skin of the fingers or hands.
   e. Warm the inunction if it will be applied to a sensitive area such as the face or back.
   f. Apply local heat to the area as ordered.
   g. Keep powders away from the nose and mouth. If they are applied near the face, do so as the patient exhales.

2. Guidelines for applying nitroglycerin ointment are (refer to page 727):
   a. Remove any previous application from the patient's skin.
   b. Squeeze a ribbon of ointment from the tube onto the manufacturer's application paper. The dosage is prescribed in centimeters or inches. The typical dosage is a 2.5- to 5-cm (1- to 2-inch) ribbon of ointment.
   c. Place the application paper containing the ribbon of ointment on a clean, nonhairy surface of the skin. The chest wall and the upper arm are usual sites.
   d. Cover the application paper with a square piece of plastic and secure with tape on four sides.
   e. Check the patient and her vital signs approximately 30 minutes after the application to determine the response of the patient.
   f. Rotate the sites on which the ointment is placed each day to prevent skin irritation.
   g. *Do not* touch the ointment. The medication can be absorbed through any skin surface.
   h. Inform the physician if the patient develops a severe headache or if there is a significant lowering of the blood pressure.

3. Common routes of topical administration for drugs are (refer to Table 33-1, page 726):
   a. Cutaneous—to the skin
   b. Sublingual—under the tongue
   c. Buccal—between the cheek and gum
   d. Vaginal—within the vagina
   e. Rectal—within the rectum
   f. Otic—within the ear
   g. Ophthalmic—within the eye
   h. Nasal—within the nose

4. For self-administration of vaginal medications, tell the patient to do the following (refer to Patient Teaching for Administering Medications Vaginally) (728):
   a. Obtain a form of medication that is to your personal preference; all come with a vaginal applicator.
   b. Plan to instill the medication before retiring for sleep to facilitate retention of the medication for a prolonged period of time.
   c. Empty your bladder just before inserting the medication.
   d. Place the drug within the applicator.
   e. Lubricate the applicator tip with a water-soluble lubricant, such as K-Y jelly.
   f. Lie down, bend your knees, and spread your legs.
   g. Separate the labia and insert the applicator within the vagina to the length recommended in the package directions, which is usually 2 to 4 inches (5–10 centimeters).
   h. Depress the plunger to insert the medication.
   i. Remove the applicator and place it on a clean tissue; discard the applicator if it is disposable.
   j. Apply a sanitary pad if you prefer.
   k. Remain recumbent for at least 10 to 30 minutes.
   l. Wash a reusable applicator when handwashing and hygiene are performed.
   m. Consult a physician if, after following the package directions, symptoms persist.

CHAPTER 34

Parenteral Medications

The number in parentheses following each rationale indicates on which page in *Fundamental Skills and Concepts in Patient Care,* Seventh Edition, you can find the correct answer.

ANSWERS TO MATCHING QUESTIONS

Items 1 Through 4

(Refer to page 741)

1. (d)
2. (b)
3. (a)
4. (c)

ANSWERS TO MULTIPLE CHOICE QUESTIONS

Items 1 Through 12

1. (a)   To ensure that the second vial will not be contaminated when combining drugs from two multiple-dose vials, the nurse should change the needle after drawing out the first medication and before inserting it into the second vial of medication. (Another method of avoiding contamination is described in Nursing Guidelines for Mixing Insulin page 743)
2. (c)   The common site for intramuscular injections into the gluteus maximus muscle is the dorsogluteal site.   (744)
3. (a)   The common site for intramuscular injections into the anterior aspect of the thigh is the rectus femoris muscle.   (744)
4. (b)   The preferred site for intramuscular injections for infants is the rectus femoris muscle. The gluteal muscles of infants are poorly developed.   (740)

5. (c)   Intramuscular injections into the deltoid muscle should be limited to 1 ml of solution and should be used only for adults.   (745)
6. (b)   One of the accepted methods for determining the dorsogluteal site to give intramuscular medications is to palpate the posterior iliac spine and the greater trochanter and draw an imaginary diagonal line between the two landmarks. The other accepted method is to divide the buttock into imaginary quadrants by drawing an imaginary vertical line through the bony ridge of the posterior superior iliac spine and an imaginary horizontal line from the upper cleft in the fold of the buttock.   (744)
7. (b)   The reason for using the Z-track technique when giving intramuscular medication is to seal the medication within the muscle so that it cannot leak back through the layers of tissue following the path of the needle.   (746)
8. (d)   A shorter needle, usually 1/2 to 5/8 inch, may be selected when giving subcutaneous injections because the tissue into which the medication will be injected is not as deep as muscular tissue. A 25-gauge needle is most often used because the medications administered by the subcutaneous route are generally not viscous.   (738)
9. (b)   Insulin is supplied in a dosage strength called a unit. The equivalent now commonly used for measuring insulin is referred to as U-100. This means that when insulin is prepared by pharmaceutical companies, the standard strength is 100 units of insulin per 1 ml.   (742)
10. (a)   Heparin is an anticoagulant. Various techniques are recommended to prevent bruising and bleeding when heparin is given via subcutaneous injection. Since heparin is also given intravenously, the nurse should not aspirate the plunger to make sure the needle is not in a vein. Drawing back on the plunger of the syringe may cause bruising or bleeding in the area of the injection.   (743)

11. (d)   The angle of the syringe and needle for intradermal injections is 10° to 15° because the medication is placed within the layers of the skin.   (750)

12. (b)   Humulin N insulin is an intermediate-acting insulin.   (743)

ANSWERS TO TRUE OR FALSE QUESTIONS

Items 1 Through 11

1. *False.* The term *parenteral* refers to all routes of administration *other* than oral.   (737)

2. *True.*

3. *False.* When combining medications from single-dose and multiple-dose vials, the medication should be withdrawn from the multiple-dose vial first.

4. *False.* An *ampule* is a glass container holding a single dose of a parenteral medication. A *vial* is a glass container of parenteral medication with a self-sealing stopper. A vial may contain one or more doses of a medication.   (738–739)

5. *False.* When giving an intramuscular injection, the needle should be inserted without hesitation. Instill the medication slowly and remove the needle rapidly to decrease the amount of medication that may spread into surrounding tissue.   (747)

6. *False.* One advantage of using prefilled cartridges is that they eliminate the time involved in transferring the drug from a medication container, like an ampule or vial, into a syringe. If the prescribed dosage is less than that contained in the cartridge, the unneeded portion is expelled before its administration to the patient.   (740)

7. *False.* Most prefilled cartridges are intended for a single-unit dose of drug.   (740)

8. *False.* When planning to administer medication via the Z-track method, the original needle used to aspirate medication into the syringe must be changed. This prevents tissue contact with residue of the drug that could be clinging to the outside of the needle.   (746)

9. *True.*

10. *True.*

11. *False.* Do not aspirate the plunger when giving heparin via the subcutaneous route.   (743)

ANSWERS TO SHORT ANSWER QUESTIONS

Items 1 Through 2

1. Criteria for selecting the appropriate syringe and needle are (refer to page 738):
   a. The *route* of administration—a longer needle is required for reaching deeper layers of tissue
   b. The *viscosity,* or thickness, of the solution—some medications are more viscous than others and require a larger lumen through which to inject the drug
   c. The *quantity* to be administered—the larger the volume of medication to be injected, the greater the holding capacity must be within the syringe
   d. The *body size* of the patient—an obese person may require a longer needle to reach various layers of tissue than a thin or pediatric patient
   e. The *type of medication*—some drugs should be measured or administered using specific equipment

2. Postneedle-stick recommendations are   (738):
   a. Report the injury to one's supervisor.
   b. Document the injury in writing.
   c. Identify the source of the blood, if known.
   d. Obtain HIV and HBV patient status results, if it is legal to do so.
   e. Obtain counseling on the potential for infection.
   f. Receive the most appropriate postexposure prophylaxis.
   g. Be tested for the presence of antibodies at appropriate intervals.
   h. Receive instructions on monitoring potential symptoms and medical follow-up.

CHAPTER 35

Intravenous Medications

The number in parentheses following each rationale indicates on which page in *Fundamental Skills and Concepts in Patient Care*, Seventh Edition, you can find the correct answer.

ANSWERS TO MATCHING QUESTIONS

Items 1 Through 5

(Refer to text in Chapter 35)

1. (e)
2. (b)
3. (c)
4. (d)
5. (a)

ANSWERS TO MULTIPLE CHOICE QUESTIONS

Items 1 Through 10

1. (d)   Medications can be added to a large volume of intravenous solution and administered slowly over a number of hours. The medication can be added to the solution by the nurse.   (757)
2. (c)   Tunneled catheters are inserted into a central vein with a portion of the catheter secured within the subcutaneous tissue. The end of the catheter exits from the skin lateral to the xiphoid process. Tunneled catheters are used when the patients require extended therapy.   (761)
3. (d)   Antineoplastic drugs are toxic to both normal and abnormal cells. It has been found that these drugs can even cause adverse effects in the pharmacists who mix them and the nurses who administer them. They can be absorbed by health care professionals through inhalation of tiny droplets or dust particles. Long-term, unprotected exposure to small amounts of these drugs can lead to changes in body cells, including sperm, ova, or fetal tissue.   (762-763)
4. (c)   There are three types of central venous catheters: percutaneous, tunneled, and implanted. The Hickman is an example of a tunneled catheter.   (766)
5. (c)   An intermittent infusion is one in which IV medication is given within a relatively short period of time.   (758)
6. (a)   Since the entire dose of medication is administered so fast, bolus administration has the greatest potential for causing life-threatening changes should a drug reaction occur.   (759)
7. (d)   One of the best features of a medication lock is that it eliminates the need for a continuous, sometimes unnecessary, administration of IV fluid.   (759)
8. (d)   A secondary infusion involves administering a drug that has been diluted in a small volume of IV solution, usually 50 to 100 cc, over a period of 30 to 60 minutes.   (760)
9. (a)   A volume-control set may be used for two purposes: to administer IV medication in a small volume at intermittent intervals and to avoid overloading the circulatory system.   (760)
10. (c)   Central venous catheters may have a single or multiple lumen. The advantage of multiple lumen is that incompatible substances, or more than one solution or drug, can be given simultaneously. Each infuses through a separate channel and exits the catheter at a different location near the heart. Thus, the drugs or solutions never interact with one another.   (761)

ANSWERS TO TRUE OR FALSE QUESTIONS

Items 1 Through 10

1. *False.* A bolus is a single dose of medication injected directly into an intravenous line. (758)
2. *False.* A heparin lock is a device that facilitates access to the bloodstream without requiring the continuous infusion of fluids. (759)
3. *True.*
4. *True.*
5. *True.*
6. *False.* Tunneled catheters are inserted into central veins and secured within subcutaneous tissue. (761)
7. *False.* A portion of many drugs is bound to protein in the blood. Drugs that are protein bound are basically inactive. That portion which is not bound is called "free drug"; it is the "free drug" that is physiologically active. Older adults tend to have more free drug in proportion to bound drug. Therefore, they are more likely to experience adverse drug effects. (764)
8. *False.* With the revocation of the Medicare Catastrophic Coverage Act of 1988, the cost of administering intravenous drugs during home care is not currently reimbursed. (770)
9. *True.*
10. *True.*

ANSWERS TO SHORT ANSWER QUESTIONS

Items 1 Through 3

(Refer to Nursing Guidelines for Administering Medications through a lock, page 759)
1. The four steps (SASH) a nurse should follow when giving medication through a heparin lock are
   a. S = Saline irrigation
   b. A = Administer medication
   c. S = Saline irrigation
   d. H = Heparin instillation

2. The advantages for using a central venous catheter over a peripheral one include (refer to pages 761-762)
   a. It avoids the necessity for multiple or frequent venipunctures when drug and fluid therapy may involve an extended length of administration.
   b. Since the catheter deposits drugs into a large blood vessel with a high volume of blood, it allows irritating or highly concentrated drugs and solutions to be instilled without traumatizing the vein wall.
   c. Some have a dual use in that venous blood can be withdrawn from the catheter rather than puncturing a peripheral vein when blood tests are ordered.
   d. A central venous catheter reduces the potential for infiltration.
   e. It frees the patient's hands for movement and self-care.

3. Intravenous administration is the route chosen when (refer to pages 757-758)
   a. A quick response is needed during an emergency.
   b. Patients have disorders that affect absorption or metabolism of drugs, such as a seriously burned patient.
   c. Blood levels of drugs need to be maintained at a consistent therapeutic level, such as when treating infections caused by drug-resistant pathogens or when providing pain relief postoperatively.
   d. It is in the patient's best interests to avoid the discomfort of repeated intramuscular injections.
   e. A mechanism is needed to administer drug therapy over a prolonged period of time, as in the case of patients with cancer.

C H A P T E R 3 6

Airway Management

The number in parentheses following each rationale indicates on which page in *Fundamental Skills and Concepts in Patient Care,* Seventh Edition, you can find the correct answer.

ANSWERS TO MATCHING QUESTIONS

Items 1 Through 5

(Refer to text in Chapter 36)

1. (e)
2. (a)
3. (b)
4. (d)
5. (c)

ANSWERS TO MULTIPLE CHOICE QUESTIONS

Items 1 Through 12

1. (c) The respiratory tract is lined with mucous membrane. This tissue keeps the passageways moist and sticky so that nongaseous particles are trapped before falling into delicate smaller structures within the lungs. Dry air or reduced volumes of water can alter the moist condition within the air passages. The mucous membranes can become dehydrated, causing mucous to become thicker than usual. To avoid this, the nurse may keep the patient well hydrated. This is done by encouraging an adequate fluid intake. (780)

2. (d) *Aerosolization* is the process of suspending droplets of water in a gas. *Humidification* is adding moisture to air; the production of rather large droplets is known as *atomization;* and *nebulization* is the production of a mist or fog. (780)

3. (b) Postural drainage should be performed before meals and before bedtime. Some positions for postural drainage are uncomfortable and may produce nausea and vomiting when therapy is carried out soon after eating. (781)

4. (a) *Percussion* is the technique of striking the chest with rhythmic gentle blows using a cupped hand. *Vibration* is the technique of using firm, strong, circular movements on the chest with open hands, producing wavelike tremors. (782)

5. (c) Percussion and vibration are intended to cause thick secretions to break loose from their location within the airway. The patient may cough up these secretions after the treatment, and collapse of the lungs possibly will be prevented by using percussion and vibration. (782)

6. (a) To determine the appropriate size of oral airway to use, place the airway on the outside of the patient's cheek; the front should be parallel with the front teeth and the back of the airway should reach the angle of the jaw. (783)

7. (c) A sputum specimen is best obtained early in the morning because a higher volume of secretions is likely to have accumulated throughout the night. Another time that may provide a better opportunity for collecting specimens would be following respiratory therapy treatments, postural drainage, and percussion and vibration. (780)

8. (d) When a patient has an oral airway in place it should be removed briefly every 4 hours. (784)

9. (b) The inner cannula of a tracheostomy should be cleaned regularly to help prevent infection. Most agencies specify that cleansing should be performed at least once every 8 hours. (783)

10. (a) When suctioning a tracheostomy, the catheter should be inserted carefully and slowly about 10 to 12.5 cm (4–5 inches) into the inner cannula and into the respiratory passage without covering the vent on the tubing. (784)

342

11. (b) Patients suffering from insufficient oxygen often feel as though they are suffocating. They are usually restless, and anxious. (Applicable Nursing Diagnoses, page 784)

12. (a) The epiglottis protects the airway by sealing the tube when swallowing food and fluids. (779 and Fig. 36-1)

ANSWERS TO TRUE OR FALSE QUESTIONS

Items 1 Through 9

1. *True.*
2. *False.* The source of suction may be through a wall unit or a separate portable machine. Usually a pressure of 100 to 140 mm Hg using a wall unit or a setting of 10 to 15 mm Hg using a portable suction machine is sufficient to remove secretions from an adult without damaging tissue severely. (Table 36-1, page 782)
3. *True.*
4. *True.*
5. *False.* Sterile technique must be followed when suctioning is performed for a patient with a tracheostomy. (Skill 36-1, page 787)
6. *False.* Collect at least a 1-to 3-ml specimen to ensure a sufficient quantity of sputum for study. (781)
7. *True.*
8. *True.*
9. *False.* Because the tracheostomy tube is below the larynx, patients are usually unable to speak or call for help. This is very frightening for most patients. Therefore, it is important that the nurse check these patients frequently and respond immediately when they signal. (784)

ANSWERS TO SHORT ANSWER QUESTIONS

Items 1 Through 2

1. The steps to follow when inserting an oral airway are (refer to Nursing Guidelines for Inserting an Oral Airway, page 783)
   a. Gather necessary supplies.
   b. Determine the appropriate size of airway to use.
   c. Wash your hands; put on clean gloves.
   d. Explain what you are going to do.
   e. Perform oral suctioning if needed.
   f. Place the patient supine; hyperextend the neck.
   g. Open patient's mouth.
   h. Insert airway halfway.
   i. Rotate airway over tongue and insert until front is flush with lips.
   j. Assess breathing.
   k. Remove airway every four hours; provide oral hygiene; clean and reinsert airway.

2. Five approaches for airway suctioning are (refer to pages 782 and 784):
   a. Nasopharyngeal
   b. Nasotracheal
   c. Oropharyngeal
   d. Oral
   e. Tracheal

CHAPTER 37

Resuscitation

The number in parentheses following each rationale indicates on which page in *Fundamental Skills and Concepts in Patient Care,* Seventh Edition, you can find the correct answer.

ANSWERS TO MULTIPLE CHOICE QUESTIONS

Items 1 Through 10

1. (c) The carotid artery is recommended for checking the pulse of an adult during CPR. The carotid artery is a large vessel and is likely to produce more obvious pulsations than could be felt at other peripheral sites on an adult. It is also the most accessible. (797)

2. (b) Before starting cardiac compressions, it is particularly important to be sure the victim is without a pulse. If a pulse is present and compressions are given, the victim may develop a potentially fatal cardiac arrhythmia. (797)

3. (c) Rescue breathing for an adult should be done every 5 seconds, each lasting 1 to 1 1/2 seconds. (799)

4. (d) When performing CPR, the ratio of compressions to ventilations should be 15 compressions to 2 ventilations. (798)

5. (c) The depth of chest compressions for an adult should be 1 1/2 to 2 inches. (798)

6. (a) Inability to sustain spontaneous ventilation is described as a state in which the response pattern of decreased energy reserves results in an individual's inability to maintain breathing adequate to support life. (799)

7. (b) For an unconscious victim, place the hands in the midline above the navel with the heel of one hand above the other and the fingers interlocked. (See Skill 37–1, page 803)

8. (c) In the presence of complete airway obstruction, the victim will be unable to speak, cough, or breathe. (796)

9. (a) The method of choice for opening the airway is the head tilt-chin lift technique. (797)

10. (b) A breathing victim is placed in the recovery position. The recovery position is a side-lying position, which helps to maintain an open airway and prevent aspiration. (797)

ANSWERS TO TRUE OR FALSE QUESTIONS

Items 1 Through 10

1. *False.* Use a brachial artery to check for a pulse in an infant. The carotid artery is recommended for use when doing CPR on an adult. (797)

2. *False.* Two rescue breaths are recommended when starting CPR on individuals of any age. (799)

3. *True.*

4. *True.*

5. *False.* It is possible to identify in an advanced directive exactly the type of resuscitation one will allow. (800)

6. *True.*

7. *True.*

8. *False.* To dislodge an object from an infant's airway, a series of back blows are delivered followed by a series of chest thrusts. (796)

9. *True.*

10. *False.* The decision to cease is a medical judgment made by the physician leading the code. (798)

ANSWERS TO SHORT ANSWER QUESTIONS

Items 1 Through 3

1. The signs of choking are (refer to pages 795–796):
   a. Grasping the throat
   b. Spontaneous efforts to cough and breathe
   c. Producing a high-pitched sound while inhaling
   d. Turning pale, then blue
   e. Being unable to speak, breathe, or cough
   f. Collapsing and becoming unconscious
2. The ABCs of basic life support are (refer to page 797):
   a. A is for airway
   b. B is for breathing
   c. C is for circulation
3. Criteria for interrupting CPR are (798):
   a. There is a pulse and the victim resumes breathing.
   b. Advanced cardiac life support measures are administered.
   c. Exhaustion of the rescuer occurs.
   d. Deterioration progresses despite resuscitation efforts.
   e. There is written evidence that resuscitation is contrary to the victim's wishes.

C H A P T E R   3 8

Death and Dying

The number in parentheses following each rationale indicates on which page in *Fundamental Skills and Concepts in Patient Care*, Seventh Edition, you can find the correct answer.

ANSWERS TO MATCHING QUESTIONS

Items 1 Through 5

(Refer to Table 38-1, page 810)

1. (c)
2. (e)
3. (a)
4. (d)
5. (b)

ANSWERS TO MULTIPLE CHOICE QUESTIONS

Items 1 Through 10

1. (c) An advanced directive is a written statement describing the wishes of the writer concerning his medical care when his death is near. (Review Chapter 3)
2. (c) The third stage of dying according to Dr. Elisabeth Kübler-Ross is the bargaining stage. (810)
3. (b) Anger is considered to be the second stage of dying. (810)
4. (c) The nurse realizes that in some instances the care needed by dying patients is too complex or demanding for family members. Families may have neither the physical nor the emotional strength to deal with the terminally ill person in the home. Care must be taken that the family is not made to feel guilty about not having the ill person at home. (812)
5. (a) Hospice care emphasizes helping the patient live until he dies, with his family with him, and helping the family return to normal living after the patient's death. (813)
6. (d) Fears are as varied as attitudes toward death. Both may change from time to time as a terminal illness progresses. Most people fear death because it represents a force over which there is no control. Generally, by relieving an individual's fears concerning death, the nurse can facilitate moving to the stage of acceptance wherein the patient can die in peace and dignity. (810)
7. (a) The patient may suck on gauze soaked in water or on ice chips wrapped in gauze without difficulty because sucking is one of the last reflexes to disappear as death approaches. (812)
8. (c) When pain is intense, relief is more difficult to obtain with the irregular administration of drugs. Therefore, it is better to try to control pain when it is minimal rather than wait until it is excruciating. Peaks and valleys of pain can be reduced by administering pain-relieving drugs on a routine schedule throughout the 24-hour period, rather than only when necessary. (813)
9. (d) The patient must be pronounced dead by the physician. At one time the patient was pronounced dead when there was no evidence of pulse, respiration, or blood pressure. In the case of extensive use of artificial means for maintaining life support, other criteria have been adopted in order to redefine death. New assessments are now used to declare individuals *brain dead*. Brain wave recordings are taken over a period of 24 hours to validate the death. (815)
10. (c) A coroner has the right to order that an autopsy be performed if the death involved a crime, was of a suspicious nature, or occurred without any medical consultation prior to the death. (815)